# Urologic Cancer

## A Multidisciplinary Perspective

# Urologic Cancer

## A Multidisciplinary Perspective

Edited by
## Marc B. Garnick, M.D.

*Dana-Farber Cancer Institute*
*Boston, Massachusetts*

and
## Jerome P. Richie, M.D.

*Brigham and Women's Hospital*
*Boston, Massachusetts*

PLENUM MEDICAL BOOK COMPANY
New York and London

Library of Congress Cataloging in Publication Data

Main entry under title:

Urologic cancer.

Includes bibliographical references.
1. Genito-urinary organs—Cancer. I. Garnick, Marc B. II. Richie, Jerome P.
[DNLM: 1. Urologic Neoplasms—Congresses. WJ 160 U78 1982]
QC280.G4U76   1983                    616.99′46                        83-17720
ISBN-13: 978-1-4684-1184-3        e-ISBN-13: 978-1-4684-1182-9
DOI: 10.1007/978-1-4684-1182-9

© 1983 Plenum Publishing Corporation
Softcover reprint of the hardcover 1st edition 1983
233 Spring Street, New York, N.Y. 10013

Plenum Medical Book Company is an imprint of Plenum Publishing Corporation

# PREFACE

The Department of Continuing Education of Harvard Medical School and members of the faculty of Harvard Medical School held a multidisciplinary course on the management of patients with urologic cancer in the fall of 1982. This course highlighted the multidisciplinary approach to the care of these patients, and outlined the clinical and pathophysiological basis for diagnosis and treatment. The term <u>multidisciplinary</u> was essential to the course in which the disciplines of urologic surgery, medical oncology, and radiation therapy were each appropriately emphasized.

Widespread interest in the contents of this course, and the timely and useful nature of much of the information presented there, has encouraged us to publish, in as rapid a manner as possible, new information and highlights of that course. A camera-ready format was used to allow rapid production, and a variety of disparate styles were maintained from chapter to chapter--some in prose, others in outline. Again, our intent was to disseminate information rapidly and accurately, and to that end, we felt that consistency of style was irrelevant.

The contents of this volume reflect the presentations of a course on the management of patients with urologic cancer, and this volume is not intended to be a comprehensive textbook on the subject. Rather, it is assumed that the readers of this volume will already have a basic foundation in the principles and practices of management of patients with urologic cancer, and that they will derive from this volume the new and exciting information that was presented in our course. We hope that this volume will contribute to more successful, multidisciplinary management of patients with urologic cancer.

Marc B. Garnick, M.D.
Jerome P. Richie, M.D.

Boston, Massachusetts

v

# ACKNOWLEDGMENT

The editors wish to express their sincere thanks to all contributors. Their diligent efforts in preparation of their manuscripts and outlines made this volume a reality. Ms. Robin Gibbs and Ms. Martha J. Sack provided unyielding patience and excellence in all aspects of management of the day-to-day editorial activities. We also wish to express our thanks to the Plenum Publishing Corporation for their encouragement throughout this project.

CONTENTS

SECTION I


PROSTATE CANCER


Prostate cancer continues to be a major public health problem. In 1983, approximately 65,000 new clinically evident cases will be diagnosed. Twenty-four thousand patients will die secondary to prostate cancer. The prompt diagnosis and optimal management is thus a major challenge to urológists, medical oncologists, and radiation therapists. This section outlines in a historical perspective the natural history and staging of prostate adenocarcinoma with a special emphasis on the heterogeneity of clinical presentations and clinical behavior. The role of the urologic oncologist in surgical management of patients with prostate cancer is discussed, followed by a dissussion of other treatment modalities. Specifically, the role of interstitial radiation therapy, external beam radiation therapy, and the more problematical circumstance in managing patients with advanced disease complement earlier sections.

CHAPTER 1

PROSTATE CANCER - NATURAL HISTORY AND STAGING

Willet F. Whitmore, Jr.


There is no universally accepted system for either the
grading or staging of prostatic neoplasms. Furthermore,
although the normal prostate is not a histologically homogeneous organ, the implications of such heterogeneity for the
histogenesis of prostatic neoplasms need better definition.
This discussion will be limited to the "acinar" adenocarcinoma
of the prostate without further references to possible differ-
ences in histogenesis. In the U.S.A., a variety of systems
for the grading of prostatic cancer has been utilized and has
been found to correlate with prognosis - the Mostofi, Gaeta,
Mayo Clinic, Bean and Gleason systems among others. Each
recognizes "good," "intermediate" and "bad" tumors, and each
suffers from an inability to consistently distinguish the
"good intermediate" from the "bad intermediate" lesions.

Relative to staging, the TNM and the American systems are
both widely used. The TNM system has the advantage of clearly
categorizing the primary tumor (T) distinct from lymph node
(N) or distant metastasis (M). The American system has the
advantage of priority and long usage, and the various subcategories that have evolved have served clinical needs well,
although definitions of the subcategories lack uniformity and
general acceptance.

Clinical staging usually includes history, physical exam,
serum acid and alkaline phosphatase, intravenous urogram and
bone scan. For better definition of the local extent of the
primary tumor, bimanual exam and cystoendoscopy under anesthesia and CT scan are useful. For clinical evaluation of
regional or juxta-regional lymph nodes, lymphangiogram, lymph-

3

oscintigraphy and CT scan, supplemented by "skinny needle" biopsy, may be employed. Surgical staging remains a common practice.

The natural history of a tumor may be defined as the clinical and pathologic manifestations of the untreated neo-plasm over time. Such characterization provides the basis of logical therapy, and logical therapy should in turn impact favorably upon it. Prostatic adenocarcinoma has an extremely varied and unpredictable natural history. This is evident from direct observations of the course of untreated prostatic cancer and from circumstantial evidence derived from observa-tions in treated patients.

The natural history can be examined in terms of two features: (1) the pattern of stage progression and (2) the growth rate. Such an analysis provides at least one logical basis for explaining the varied behavior of the disease. Although it seems almost inevitable that host factors influence tumor behavior, the absence of data precludes intel-ligent discussion of the latter possibility at this time.

I. STAGE PROGRESSION

   A--------→   B---------→   C---------→   D

Such a pattern of stage progression is simple, not illogi-cal, clearly desirable from the standpoint of therapy, and highly optimistic

Clinical and pathologic evidence, largely assembled over the past 10 years, have, however, indicated that a variety of other patterns of progression are possible:

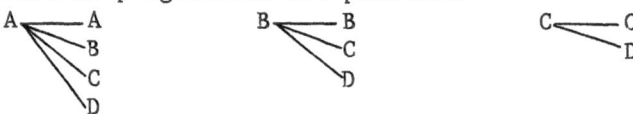

Given groups of patients with stage A, B or C prostatic cancer, the frequency with which the different potential patterns of stage progression occur is still incompletely defined, and this lack of definition is more evident the earl-ier the stage. Furthermore, in an individual patient, prog-nostication of behavior is currently impossible. Thus, the earlier the tumor stage, the greater the possibilities of

tumor behavior and the more difficult the task of recom-
mending therapy and of evaluating the impact of the therapy
per se upon the subsequent clinical course.

In practical terms the metastatic potential of a prostatic cancer is positively indicated only by the identification of metastasis, and clinical staging techniques and
staging lymphadenectomy are performed to determine whether
this potential has been manifested.

## II. GROWTH RATE

The growth rate of a tumor is a complex function of the
intermitotic interval, the relative proportions of cycling and
non-cycling cells, cell death, and tumor size. Although it
can be represented by more sophisticated models, for present
purposes the general significance of growth rate to the proli-
feration of a solid tumor can be represented in a fashion
which disregards cell death, non-cycling cells and size.

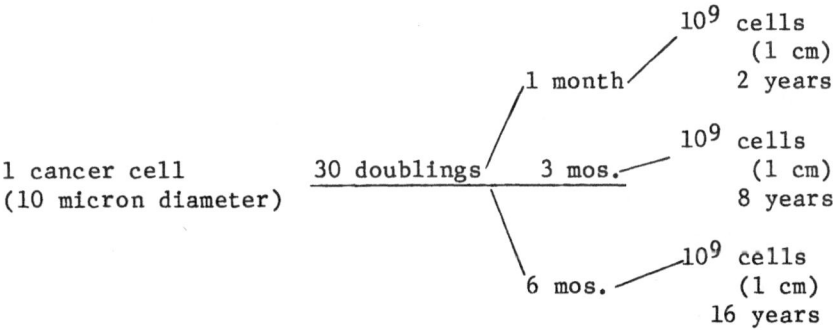

Estimations of tumor doubling times may be derived from
tritiated thymidine labelling indices (TLI) which utilize
radioautographic detection of labelled DNA as an indication of
the proportion of cells in DNA as an indication of the porpor-
tion of cells in DNA synthesis (cycling cells), or from actual
physical measurements of tumor size over time. For prostatic
cancers, such information is limited but is in accord with the
possibility that some prostatic tumors have doubling times of
the order of 6 months. For practical purposes, however, one
must recognize that in seeing a patient at a single point in
time, one has no simple and reliable way of estimating growth
rate. TLI is not a practical test even if it were totally

reliable.   Serial observations with time give some indication
of growth rate but are obviously not uniformly practical in
the clinical situtation.

Tumor grade as assessed by conventional light microscopy correlates in a general way both with pattern of stage
progression and with growth rate and is the best practical
measure we currently have, but we clearly need something
better.   Tumor cell heterogeneity involves the concept that
morphologically similar tumors differ remarkably in behavior,
and morphologically similar cells (at least as determined by
conventional light microscopy)  within a single tumor may have
enormously different biologic potentials.

The existence of two more of less independent (and largely
unquantifiable variables) within a given prostatic cancer -
pattern of stage progression and growth rate - contribute to
the present uncertainty regarding management of prostatic
cancer.

SELECTED REFERENCES

1. Murphy, G.P. and Whitmore, W.F., Jr.:  A report of the
   workshops on the current status of the histologic grading
   of prostatic cancer.   Cancer 44:1490, 1979.

2. Franks, L.M. and Durh, M.B.: Latency and progression in
   tumours.   The natural history of prostatic cancer.   Lancet
   17:1037, 1956.

3. Franks, L.M., Fergusson, J.D., and Murnaghan, G.F.:  An
   assessment of factors influencing survival in prostatic
   cancer:  The absence of reliable prognostic features.
   Brit. J. Cancer 12:321, 1958.

4. Gleason, D.F.:  Classification of prostatic carcinomas.
   Cancer Chemother. Rep. 5:125, 1966.

5. McNeal, J.E.:  Anatomy of the prostate:  An historical
   survey of divergent views.   The Prostate 1:3, 1980.

6. Whitmore, W.F., Jr.:  The natural history of prostatic
   cancer.   Cancer 32:1104, 1973.

7. Prout, G.R., Jr.: Diagnosis and staging of prostatic carcinoma Cancer 32:1096, 1973.

8. Fowler, J.E., Jr. and Whitmore, W.F., Jr.: The incidence and extent of pelvic lymph node metastases in apparently localized prostatic cancer. Cancer 47:2941, 1981.

9. Mostofi, F.K.: Problems of grading carcinoma of prostate. Semin. Oncol. 3:161, 1976.

10. Franks, L.M.: The spread of prostatic cancer. J. Path. & Bacteriol. 157:603, 1956.

11. Baserga, R.: The cell cycle. N. Eng. J. Med. 304:453, 1981.

12. Whitehead, E.D. and Leiter, E.: Prostatic carcinoma. Clincial and surgical staging. New York State J. Med. 2:184, 1981.

13. Fidler, I.J. and Kripke, M.L.: Metastasis results from preexisting variant cells within a malignant tumor. Science 197:893, 1977.

14. Fidler, I.J. and Hart, I.R.: The origin of metastatic heterogeneity in tumors. Europ. J. Cancer 17:487, 1981.

15. McCullough, D.L.: Surgical staging of carcinoma of the prostate. Cancer 45:1902, 1980.

16. Murphy, G.P., et al.: Current status of classification and staging of prostate cancer. Cancer 45:1889, 1980.

CHAPTER 2

SURGICAL MANAGEMENT OF PROSTATE CANCER

Lester Klein

I.  PROSTATE BIOPSY

Usually done by needle, but TUR-biopsy and open biopsy are alternative techniques.

A.  INDICATIONS

1.  Suspicious nodule:

a.  KUB should be obtained to exclude calcification, which may feel like a "hard mass."

b.  50% of "nodules" are not cancer.  Granulomas, calculi and dense stomal hypertrophy should be considered.

c.  "Negative" biopsy, i.e., failure to obtain any prostate tissue or only normal prostate tissue, must be repeated either by the same method or by another operative approach (e.g., open biopsy).

d.  "Nodule of BPH" may be an adequate pathological explanation but acceptance of this finding depends on the certainty of the surgeon that the suspicious lesion was actually sampled.

2. To confirm the diagnosis of prostate cancer when acid phosphatase and bone scan are positive and prostate feels hard. The necessity of "tissue diagnosis" should be evaluated since treatment may be offered in some circumstances even without histological diagnosis.

B. TECHNIQUES

1. Perineal: done by passing a biopsy needle percutaneously via the perineum to the prostate, guiding the needle to the nodule by a finger in the rectum.

   a. Preparation--general anesthesia (or spinal) is usually suggested. Bleeding and clotting time should be normal. Systemic antibiotics are optional. Cystoscopy may be done at the termination of procedure to evaluate bleeding and need for catheter drainage.

   b. Advantages--avoids rectal perforation (see below). No need for antibiotic enema.

   c. Complications--bleeding, urinary retention (less than 5%). Failure to diagnose ranges from about 5% in the presence of large clinical lesions to 50% for nodules.

2. Transrectal biopsy: done by passing a skinny needle or Frantze aspiration needle through the anus and perforating the rectal mucosa at the level of prostate.

   a. Preparation--antibiotics by enema and systemically. Hematological evaluation less important since bleeding is uncommon.

   b. Advantages--outpatient procedure, avoids anesthesia, reduces failure to diagnose to 20% when problem is a nodule.

   c. Complications--Urosepsis has been reported.

3. TUR Biopsy: done with a resectoscope.

a.  Preparation--general or spinal anesthesia,
    hematological evaluation.

b.  Advantages--Corrects urinary obstruction if
    present. May be positive if needle biopsy
    negative.

c.  Disadvantages--may make subsequent treatment
    more difficult. May spread the neoplasm. TUR
    biopsy, compared to needle biopsy, exhibits an
    increase in recurrence rate (local or distal)
    from 24% to 50% (p=.001) and a death rate
    which increases from 18% to 34% (p=.001).
    This detrimental effect is independent of
    tumor size or grade. The data which is the
    basis for those statements derives from a
    retrospective analysis. It is unclear if the
    patients diagnosed by needle biopsy are really
    comparable to those diagnosed by TUR. More
    date is needed to determine if the observation
    is realistic.

II. LYMPHADENECTOMY

This diagnostic test examines the obturator and iliac
lymph nodes and is not considered to be therapeutic.

A.  Staging of prostatic cancer begins with the non-
    invasive studies of acid phosphatase, bone survey and
    bone scan. If these tests are all negative (normal),
    then an evaluation of the prostatic regional lymph
    nodes is needed to determine "curability." Methods
    available for lymph node assessment are (1) lymphan-
    giography, (2) lymphoscintigraphy, (3) needle biopsy
    under fluoroscopic control, (4) CT scan and (5) lymph
    node biopsy. The last is the "gold standard" in
    accuracy. The first four options are not as accurate
    as open lymphadenectomy.

B.  Lymphadenectomy has no false positives. This compares
    well to acid phosphatase false positive rate of
    40-70%. Fifty percent of patients with high-grade
    lesions using Gleason histological staging have
    negative nodes. The percent of false positives, i.e.,
    high grade lesion without involved lymph nodes,

depends on the stage of cancer determined by digital
rectal examination.

False negatives do occur with lymphadenectomy, especially when frozen sections are utilized.  False
negative rates may be decreased by limiting biopsy to
the obturator nodes.  These are the primary draining
nodes and so have the highest potential yield of
malignancy.  With obturator nodes only, the patholo-
gist has less material to examine and so may do a more
thorough examination.

C.  Technique

Because the procedure is for biopsy, any suspicious
nodes should be sought and excised before an extensive
dissection is done.  Obturator nodes should be
obtained from the ipsilateral side initially and that
tissue examined before completing the contralateral
side.  The procedure should be extraperitoneal in
order to avoid adhesions of bowel to pelvis with
subsequent increased risk of radiation-induced
enteritis.  Care should be taken to avoid cutting
lymphatics without ligature control in order to reduce
risk of lymphocoele.

D.  Complications

Overall, the rate of complications may be 20%,
although, death is rare (less than 0.5%).  Lymphocoeles of clinical significance occur in 5% of
patients and pulmonary emboli in 2%.

E.  Postoperative care

Anticoagulation is debatable because the increased
incidence of lymphocoeles may balance the decreased
incidence of pulmonary embolization.


III.  RADICAL PROSTATECTOMY

This procedure consists of the removal of the prostate
gland including its capsule, the ejaculatory ducts,
seminal vesicles and the ventral layer of Denonvilliers
fascia.  A urethral-vesical anastomosis is required.

A.  INDICATIONS

The neoplasm must be localized to the gland (Stage A
or B).  In theory, a neoplasm which extends through
the capsule (Stage C) could be cured by operation but
experience shows that to be infrequent.  The patient
should be less than 70 years old and in good general
health, i.e., he should have a normal life expectancy
of over 10 years.

B.  TECHNIQUES

1.  Perineal-the "classical" approach
    a.  Advantages: ease of exposure for excision and for
        urethral-vesical anastomosis.
    b.  Disadvantages:  does not permit examination of
        lymph nodes as part of the procedure.
2.  Retropubic--a more recent development
    a.  Advantages:  may be done in connection with lymph
        node sampling.  Many urologists are more familiar
        with the anatomic planes associated with this
        operation.
    b.  Disadvantages:  The incision is more painful than
        the perineal.  The incidence of pulmonary and
        phlebitic problems may be higher.

C.  COMPLICATIONS

1.  Impotency--recent experience based upon careful
    anatomic study suggests the rate of impotency may be
    50-67%.
2.  Incontinence--about 5-10%.  The rate is unrelated to
    prior TUR prostate.

D.  RESULTS

1.  Stage $A_1$:  these patients probably survive normally
    without radical treatment.
2.  Stage $A_2$:  if there is no evidence of spread to
    nodes ("true $A_2$"), treatment with radical prosta-
    tectomy results in normal survival rates.
3.  Stage $B_1$:  15 year survival with no evidence of
    disease is 33%.
4.  Stage $B_2$:  15 year survival with no evidence of
    disease is 18%.

   5.  Overall, the incidence of local recurrence of prosta-
       tic cancer after radical prostatectomy is 13%.


IV.  ANTERIOR EXENTERATION

   This procedure consists of removal of the prostate and
   associated structures as in radical prostatectomy but
   bladder and proximal urethra also removed.  Urinary
   diversion required.

   A.  INDICATION

       1.  Large Stage B and Stage C lesions
           a.  Experience with this procedure applied to
               prostate cancer is limited.  The concept of
               "salvage" prostatectomy has not been applied
               to prostate cancer
           b.  In absence of positive nodes, cure may
               approach 67%.
       2.  Transitional cell cancer of prostate may occur
           alone or in conjunction with prostatic adenocar-
           cinoma.  May be associated with in situ bladder
           cancer.  Often found with osteolytic bone
           metastases.
           a.  TUR and total prostatectomy not curative in
               any series
           b.  Radical cystoprostatectomy yields a 55% 5 year
               survival rate.

   B.  RESULTS

       1.  Local control:  theoretically an anterior
           exenteration should be superior but small series
           fail to show better control than radical prosta-
           tectomy.  Perhaps the operation is applied too
           late in the course of the neoplasm.
       2.  Survival:  insufficient data available to comment.


V.  PALLIATIVE OPERATIONS

   A.  Orchiectomy

       1.  For advanced carcinoma.  The question of timing of
           procedure is debatable.  70% of previously

untreated patients respond well, i.e., symptoms
and/or acid phosphatase improve. 90% of men with
ureteral obstruction improve. From relapse of
symptoms after hormonal treatment to time of death
is about 10 months.

2. Options:  estrogen treatment (See Chapter 5).

B.  Adrenalectomy, Hypophysectomy

Theoretical basis is ablation of residual sources of
androgen after orchiectomy. Empirical data shows
little benefit from these procedures.

C.  Spinal cord decompression after vertebral collapse due
to metastases may save a patient from becoming a
paraplegic.

VI. SUMMARY OF SURGICAL INTERVENTION IN THE TREATMENT OF
PROSTATE CANCER--STAGE-BY-STAGE:

$A_1$    No treatment required.

$A_2$    Radical prostatectomy after thorough staging
effort. Because some feel that radiation therapy
may be effective here, radiation therapy and
prostatectomy are to be compared in a prospective
study sponsored by the National Prostate Cancer
Project.

$B_1$    Radical prostatectomy--age matched controls
survive no better than this group.

$B_2$    Radical prostatectomy, but nodes must be proven
negative.

C       Anterior exenteration--50% survival if nodes are
negative.

D       Palliative surgery only.

SELECTED REFERENCES

1.  Catalona, W.J. and Scott, W.W.: Carcinoma of the prostate:
A review. J. Urol.  119:1,1978.

2.  Klein, L.A.:  Prostate cancer. New Eng. J. Med  300: 824, 1979.

3.  Murphy, G.P., et al.:  Current status of classification and staging of prostate cancer.  Cancer 45: 1880, 1980.

4.  Walsh, P.C.:  Radical prostatectomy for the treatment of localized prostatic cancer. Urol. Clinics N. Amer. 7: 583 1980.

5   Pontes, J., et al.:  Estrogen receptors and clinical correlation with human prostatic disease Urology, 19:399, 1982.

6.  Melograna, F., et al.:  Fine needle prostatic aspiration, Urology 19:47, 1982.

7.  Catalona, W.J.:  Accuracy of frozen section detection of lymph node metastases in prostatic carcinoma, J. Urol. 127:460, 1982.

CHAPTER 3

## INTERSTITIAL RADIATION THERAPY FOR MANAGEMENT OF LOCALIZED PROSTATE CANCER

William U. Shipley

The initial reports of the clinical efficacy of inter-stitial radiotherapy for prostate cancer appeared many decades ago in the urological literature. Prior to the availability of supravoltage external beam equipment, radioactive implant techniques offered unique dose advantages for these deep-seated tumors as reported by Young in 1922, Barringer in 1942 and Flocks in 1959. However during the 1960's supravoltage external beam radiation therapy (XRT) became recognized as the treatment of choice in many patients with tumors unsuitable for resection. This was largely due to the reports from Stanford University of a large series that indicted such treatment was well tolerated, locally effective and associated with low complication rate and the preservation of sexual potency in approximately 60% of patients.

Beginning over a decade ago, Whitmore and Hilaris at the Memorial Sloan-Kettering Cancer Center and Carlton and Hudgins at the Baylor College of Medicine extended the combined surgical/radiotherapeutic role in the treatment of men with prostatic cancer by combining pelvic lymphadenectomy with the retropubic implantation of radioactive seeds. Because the radiation strategy, the radioisotope used, and some clinical indications differ at these two large American centers, I will review these experiences separately and subsequently outline some general clinical guidelines.

IODINE-125 SEED IMPLANTS

The treatment of patients with permanent interstitial
Iodine-125 radioactive seeds was developed by the Memorial
group.  Their promising results in patients with localized
prostatic carcinoma prompted many other Institutions to
initiate similar treatment programs.  Relative to other
available implant radionuclides (Iridium-192, Radon-222 or
Gold-198), the soft gamma and x-ray (27 to 35 kiloelectron
volts) radiations of Iodine-125 offer important advantages in
personal radiation safety and in reducing the dose to normal
tissue adjacent to the implanted volume.  The Memorial
strategy is that the implant delivers the full tumoricidal
radiation dose.  Because the half-life of Iodine-125 is long
(60 days), the dose-rate is low (initially 8 rads/hr).  The
total dose (16,000 rads), determined by the amount of radioactivity implanted, is absorbed over many months and is
thought to be the biologic equivalent of about 7000 rads given
with conventional external beam techniques.

Intra-operative techniques will be highlighted because an
homogeneous Iodine-125 implant is difficult at this site.
Satisfactory dose distribution in prostatic implants are
especially critical for local tumor control because 1) the
dose immediately outside the implanted volume decreases very
rapidly and 2) Iodine-125 is used to deliver the total therapeutic tumor dose, rather than as a "boost" in addition to
4000 to 5000 rads of conventional radiation, which is the
usual practice for other implant sites, such as the tongue,
breast, cervix, skin or prostate by the Baylor approach.

The results from the large series at Memorial for
patients with stages T1 (B1), T2 (B2-3) and minimal T3 tumors
are comparable to those with conventional radiation: clinical
local control, 80-95%, 5 and 10 year survivals of 80% and
50%.  However, the local control in the 65 stage T3 patients
was only 68%.

Dr. Whitmore has outlined the criteria used currently at
Memorial for Iodine-125 implants as: 1) life expectancy of 5
years or more, 2) clinical stage B or small C tumors not
extending to the seminal vesicles or to the pelvic side walls,
3) the ability to define digitally apparent margins of the
tumor, and 4) good mobility of the gland and no significant
outlet obstruction at endoscopy (5).  Most institutions doing
Iodine-125 implants are following the general Memorial
strategy.  Radiation dysuria is delayed for 2-3 months after
the implant, usually lasts 1-3 months, and is more common
(30-50%) than with external beam XRT.  Maintenance of sexual

potency is reported by 80-90% of treated patients.
Incontinence is rare.  Post-implant external beam XRT should
not be combined with this implant because the additive radiation effects will likely exceed either rectal or urologic
tolerance.

Presently, we recommend low-dose preoperative irradiation (1050 rads in 3 days to prevent possible tumor seeding),
pelvic lymphadenectomy (limited to the distal hypogastric,
obturator and medial external iliac groups) and Iodine-125
implantation as a treatment option for men with differentiated
tumors stage T2 or less, who are strongly motivated to maintain sexual potency and who do not have evidence of lymph node
metastases on surgical exploration.

COMBINED GOLD-198 SEED IMPLANT AND EXTERNAL BEAM XRT

For over 15 years the Baylor group have combined external
beam XRT (4000 to 5000 rads) with lymphadenectomy and prostatic tumor implantation of Gold-198 (2500 to 3500 rads),
with the rationale of minimizing complications while providing
a high, and thus likely curative, dose of radiation to the
tumor.  This large series has recently been updated.  The
favorable results reported (vida infra) may have been
influenced because many of 542 treated patients were excluded
from the updated survival analysis because either no pretreatment bone scan was obtained, hormonal therapy was given prior
to relapse or the clinical stage was greater than $C_1$ (6 cm).
Complications were low in all categories (i.e. transient leg
edema 10%, persistent edema 1%; potency was satisfactory in
60% of patients from 1 to 11 years following implant).  The 5
and 10 year survivals of the 232 patients (stage $A_2$, 39;
$B_1$, 36; $B_2$, 66; $C_1$, 91) were 90% and 68%, respectively.
Only 11% have developed clinical evidence of local recurrence.
Prostatic biopsies were performed between 6 and 36 months
post-implant in 129 patients with no clinical evidence of
tumor.  Seventy-nine or 61% of these patients had persis-
tently negative biopsies.  Of the 50 with a positive biopsy
only 12% have developed clinical evidence of local recurrence.

Carlton and associates recommend this approach for men
with stage $A_2$, $B_2$, $C_1$ tumors and those with stage $B_1$
who are not medically suitable or prefer not to accept the
risks and complications of radical prostatectomy.

GUIDELINES FOR RADIOACTIVE SEED IMPLANTS IN PATIENTS WITH
PROSTATIC CANCER

1.  Avoid implanting patients with significant outlet
    obstruction; if obstruction is minimal the implant
    should follow, by at least 6 weeks, a "limited TURP"
2.  Close intraoperative collaboration by the surgeon,
    radiation therapist and radiation physicist should
    prevent errors in tumor dosage; the prostatic implant
    is technically more difficult than those commonly
    done by the radiation therapist.
3.  Iodine-125 is safer than Gold-198 with respect to
    radiation protection because of its very soft gamma
    and x-ray radiations.
4.  Gold-198 is safer than Iodine-125 to combine with
    4000 to 5000 rads external beam XRT postoperatively
    because its short half-life prevents irradiation
    simultaneously by both techniques.
5.  The Gold-198 implant should only be used as a "boost"
    dose combined with 4000 to 5000 rads conventional
    XRT.
6.  For any tumor larger than a small C(T3), but smaller
    than 6 cm diameter, only the Gold-198 implant plus
    4000 to 5000 rads is an accepted implant strategy.
7.  When comparable groups (by tumor stage, histology and
    nodal status) are considered, local control, compli-
    cation rates and survival are apparently similar for
    the two implant approaches and external beam XRT by
    multiple contoured fields.
8.  Radioactive interstitial implant strategies should
    consider incorporating some preoperative XRT to
    minimize the possibility of tumor seeding.

SELECTED REFERENCES

1.  Barringer, B.S.: Prostatic carcinoma.  J. Urol. 47:306,
    1942.

2.  Barzell, W., et al.:  Prostatic adenocarcinoma:
    relationship of grade and local extent to the pattern of
    metastases.  J. Urol. 118:278, 1977.

3.  Carlton, C.E. Jr., et al.:  Irradiation treatment of
    carcinoma of the prostate.  J. Urol. 108:924, 1972.

4.    Flocks, R.H., et al.:  The treatment of carcinoma of the
      prostate by interstitial radiation with radioactive gold.
      J. Urol. 71:628, 1959.

5.    Gilbert, E.H. and Pistenma, D.A. eds.:  Workshop on the
      treatment of prostatic cancer.  National Cancer
      Institute, November 17-18, 1980.

6.    Ray, G.R., Cassidy, J.R. and Bagshaw, M.A.:  Definitive
      radiation therapy of carcinoma of the prostate.
      Radiology 106:407, 1973.

7.    Scardino, P.T., Guerriero, W.G. and Carlton, C.E. Jr.:
      Surgical staging and combined therapy with gold-198 grain
      implantation and external irradiation.  In: Johnson, D.E.
      and M.A. Boileau, M.A., eds. Genitourinary Tumors:
      General Principles and Surgical Techniques.   New York:
      Grune and Stratton, 1982, p. 75.

8.    Shipley, W.U., et al.: Preoperative irradiation,
      lymphadenectomy and Iodine-125 implant for patients with
      localized prostatic carcinoma.  J. Urol. 124:639, 1980.

9.    Whitmore, W.F.Jr., Hilaris, B.S. and Grabstand, H.:
      Retropublic implantation of Iodine-125 in the treatment
      of prostatic cancer. J. Urol. 108:918, 1972.

10.   Young, H.H.: Technique of radium treatment of cancer of
      the prostate and seminal vesicles.  Surg. Gynecol.
      Obstet. 34:93, 1922.

CHAPTER 4

EXTERNAL BEAM IRRADIATION FOR CARCINOMA OF PROSTATE

J. Robert Cassady

I.   DEMOGRAPHIC DATA

A.   Approximately 65,000 new cases/year in the United
     States.
B.   Second in incidence to lung cancer for males.
C.   Approximately 20,000 deaths/year in the United
     States.
D.   Of all cases:
     1.   50+% have overt non-nodal metastases at
          presentation.
     2.   10% have early stage (A1, B1) disease with
          favorable histology.
     3.   Around 40% have regionally extensive disease but
          no overt metastases.

II.  PRETREATMENT EVALUATION

     (in addition to history and physical exam)
A.   <u>Necessary</u>

     1.   Isotopic bone scan - essential staging procedure;
          rule out false positive scans.
     2.   Chest PA & lateral x-rays with selected bone
          x-rays
     3.   Serum prostatic acid phosphatase (SPAP) - often
          poor sensitivity and reliability.  Fractionated
          serum alkaline phosphatase.

   B.  Optional

      1.  Computerized tomography:  Of potential value in
          evaluation of loco/regional disease extent and
          for treatment planning.
      2.  Lymphangiography controversial.
      3.  Lymph node sampling (See also Chapter 2).


III.  STAGING

Table 4-1.  TNM Classification for Carcinoma of the Prostate
(Reproduced with permission, J.B. Lippincott, Company,
Philadelphia, Ref. 6)

---

Primary Tumor (T)
   TX   Minimum requirements cannot be met
   T0   No tumor palpable; includes incidental findings of cancer in a biopsy or operative specimen.
        Assign all such cases a G, N, or M category
   T1   Tumor intracapsular surrounded by normal gland
   T2   Tumor confined to gland, deforming contour, and invading capsule, but lateral sulci and
        seminal vesicles are not involved
   T3   Tumor extends beyond capsule with or without involvement of lateral sulci and/or seminal
        vesicles
   T4   Tumor fixed or involving neighboring structures. Add suffix (m) after "T" to indicate
        multiple tumors (e.g., T2m)
Nodal Involvement (N)
   NX   Minimum requirements cannot be met
   N0   No involvement of regional lymph nodes
   N1   Involvement of a single regional lymph node
   N2   Involvement of multiple regional lymph nodes
   N3   Free space between tumor and fixed pelvic wall mass
   N4   Involvement of juxta-regional nodes
   *Note:* If N category is determined by lymphangiography or isotope scans, insert "1" or "i" between
   "n" and appropriate number (e.g., N12 or Ni2). If nodes are histologically positive after surgery,
   add " +," if negative, add " −."

Distant Metastasis (M)
   MX   Not assessed
   M0   No (known) distant metastasis
   M1   Distant metastasis present
        Specify _____
        Specify sites according to the following notations:
                    Pulmonary—PUL                    Bone Marrow—MAR
                    Osseous—OSS                         Pleura—PLE
                    Hepatic—HEP                          Skin—SKI
                    Brain—BRA                              Eye—EYE
            Lymph Nodes—LYM                          Other—OTH
   *Note:* Add " +" to the abbreviated notation to indicate that the pathology (p) is proved.

A.  Pathologic and clinical extent of disease

    1.  25% of all patients with clinical B lesions will
        have pathologically involved lymph nodes.
    2.  60-70% of all patients with clinical stage C
        lesions will have pathologically involved lymph
        nodes.
    3.  30% of favorably selected patients with clinical
        stage B disease will have pathologic stage C
        disease.
    4.  A combination of histologic grade, clinical
        stage, and SPAP highly predictive for lymph node
        involvement:
        - Less than 10% + lymph nodes - grade 1-2,
        clinical stage $A_1$ or $B_1$, normal SPAP.
        - Greater than 90% + lymph nodes - grade 3,
        clinical stage C, elevated SPAP.
        - Intermediate (20-50%) + lymph nodes - any
        patient with 1 or 2 adverse features.

B.  Lymph Node Sampling and/or Dissection (See Table 4-2)

    1.  No study confirming curative potential.  Barzell
        study demonstrated long-term disease-free
        survival (not necessarily synonymous with cure)
        in patients with small volumes of nodal
        involvement.  Pearson study indicates therapy
        almost always palliative.
    2.  Useful only if therapy will modified; i.e.
        elimination of radiation therapy, introduction of
        adjuvant chemotherapy (clinical trial) or in
        combination with interstitial implantation.

IV.  EXTERNAL BEAM TREATMENT

A.  Radical (Curative) intent

    1.  No overt distant metastases.
    2.  No major pelvic or any para-aortic nodal disease.
    3.  Age generally less than 75 years.
    4.  $A_1$ patients, especially those with grade 1
        lesions, excluded.

Table 4-2.   Relationship of Gleason Pattern with Nodal
Metastatic Disease (Reproduced with permission, Williams and
Wilkins Company, Baltimore).

### Comparison of Gleason Sum with Node Biopsy

| GLEASON SUM | NODE BIOPSY | | | |
|---|---|---|---|---|
| | Positive | Negative | N/Group | |
| 2–5 | 13.9% | 86.1% | 36 | |
| 6 | 32.4% | 67.6% | 34 | |
| 7 | 49.9% | 50.1% | 21 | $X^2 = 28.2$ |
| 8 | 75.0% | 25.0% | 12 | p .0005 |
| 9–10 | 100.0% | 0% | 7 | |
| No Diagnosis | 33.3% | 66.7% | 12 | |

(Modified from Paulson DF, Piserchia PV, Gardner W: Predictions of lymphatic spread in prostatic adenocarcinoma: Uro-oncology Research Group study. J Urol 123:697–699, 1980)

### Comparison of Gleason Patterns as a Predictor of Nodal Metastatic Disease

| PELVIC LYMPHADENECTOMY | NO. PTS. | GLEASON PATTERNS | | |
|---|---|---|---|---|
| | | (2, 3, 4) | (5, 6, 7) | (8, 9, 10) |
| Positive | 53 | $\frac{0}{31}$ (0%) | $\frac{26}{84}$ (31%) | $\frac{27}{29}$ (93%) |
| Negative | 91 | $\frac{31}{31}$ (100%) | $\frac{58}{84}$ (69%) | $\frac{2}{29}$ (7%) |

(Modified from Kramer SA, Spahr J, Brendler CB, et al: Experience with Gleason Histopathologic Grading in Prostatic Cancer. J Urol 124:223–225, 1980)

Therefore, patients with:
$A_1$ – moderately or poorly differentiated
$A_2$, B1, $B_2$
are eligible

## B.   Palliative Intent

Any patient with local perineal pain, prostatic urinary tract
obstruction, or pelvic lymphatic obstruction non-responsive to
endocrine manipulation.

## C.   Technique

6000–7000 (TD max. ) rad/7-8 week by rotational (360 degrees,
120 degreees lat. arcs) or multiple (greater than 2) field

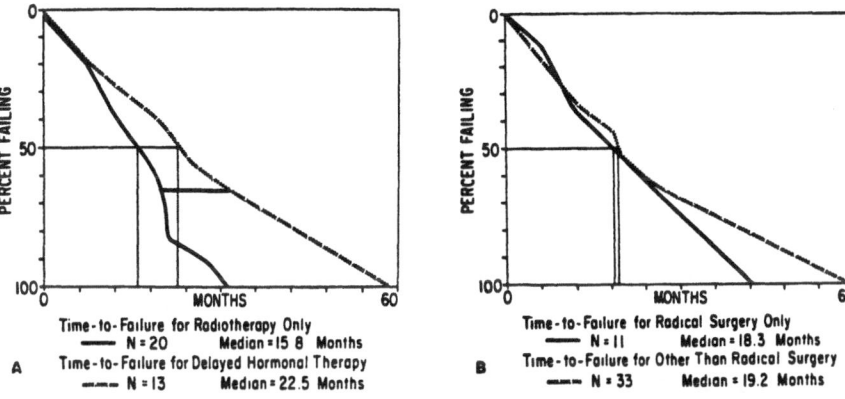

Figure 4-1. Results of treatment of patients with prostatic carcinoma and regional lymph node metastases. (Reproduced with permission, Williams and Wilkins Company, Baltimore, Ref. 7).

megavoltage portals. Fraction size/day = 150-200 rad. Initial 4000-5000 rad usually delivered to larger volume (100-150 sq. cm. field area) followed by small field (50-75 sq. cm.) boost.

D.   Results

1.   Survival

| Stage | 5 yr. | 10 yr. |
|-------|-------|--------|
| A | 100% | ? |
| B | 70-80% | 50% |
| C | 50%-55% | 30-35% |

2.   Stage Clinical local control Time to tumor regression

| Stage | Clinical local control | Time to tumor regression |
|-------|------------------------|--------------------------|
| B | 90-95% | completion - 3 mo. |
| C | 80-85% | 3-6 mo. |

Addition of estrogen therapy either before XRT or concurrent with or shortly after XRT confers no advantage and may be disadvantageous.

E.   Post-treatment biopsy

1.   Only warranted as a routine for experimental study or
     if additional local therapy contemplated (radical
     prostatectomy or interstitial implant - see Goffinet
     et al.:  Cancer 45:2717, 1980).
2.   No definite correlation established between
     post-treatment biopsy and ultimate clinical course.
3.   Nearly all patients will have a positive biopsy at
     completion of treatment, but incidence of positive
     biopsies will steadily decrease for 3-5 years after
     treatment.

F.   Complications

1.   Impotency - 30-50%
2.   Acute diarrhea/cystitis - great than 50%
3.   Chronic bowel complaints - 5-10%, depending on
     severity required and volume of XRT field
4.   Urethral stricture approximately 3% - increased with
     prior TUR, especially if XRT begun less than 4-6
     weeks after TURP.  Increased with maximum tumor doses
     over 4500.

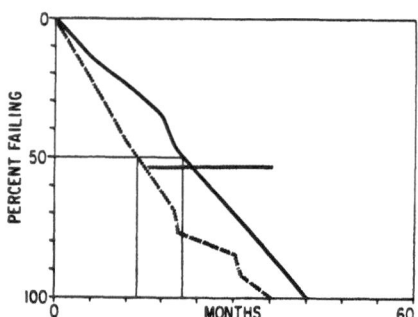

Time-to-Treatment Failure for Patients with One Positive Node
——— N = 17        Median = 21 5  Months
Time-to-Treatment Failure for Patients with More Than One
Positive Node
——— N = 18        Median = 13.7  Months

Figure 4-2.   Influence of the number of metastases on time to
treatment failure in patients with prostatic carcinoma.
(Reproduced with permission, Williams and Wilkins Company,
Baltimore, Ref. 7).

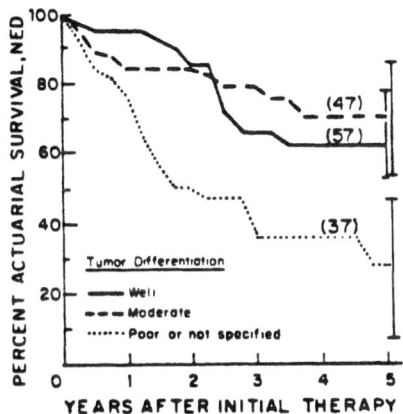

Figure 4-3. Carcinoma of Prostate – Stage C (MIR, 1966–1976)
Survival and Histological Differentation. Tumor-free
actuarial survival in patients with Stage C carcinoma of the
prostate according to histological differentiation of the
tumor. (Reproduced with permission, J.B. Lippincott Company,
Philadelphia, Ref. 6).


SELECTED REFERENCES

1.   Ray, G.R., Cassady, J.R. and Bagshaw, M.A.:  Definitive
     radiation therapy of carcinoma of the prostate.
     Radiology 106:407, 1973.

2.   Pilepich, M.V., Perez, C.A. and Bauer, W.:  Prognostic
     parameters in radiotherapeutic management of localized
     carcinoma of the prostate.  J. Urol.  124:485, 1980.

3.   Neglia, W.J., Hussey, D.H. and Johnson, D.E.:
     Megavoltage radiation therapy for carcinoma of the
     prostate.  Int. J. Rad. Oncol.  2:873, 1977.

4.   Pistenma, D.A., Ray, G.R. and Bagshaw, M.A.:  The role of
     megavoltage radiation therapy in the treatment of
     prostatic carcinoma.  Semin. Oncol.  3:115, 1976.

5.   Carlton, C.E., Jr.:  Radiotherapy in the management of
     Stage C carcinoma of the prostate.  J. Urol.  116:206,
     1976.

6.   Paulson, D.F., Perez, C.A. and Anderson, T.: Genito-
     urinary malignancies. In: Devita, V., Hellman, S. and
     Rosenberg, S.A., eds. Principles and Practice of
     Oncology. Philadelphia: Lippincott, 1982, pp. 732-779.

7.   Kramer, S.A., Cline, W.A., Jr., Farnham, R., et.al.:
     Prognosis of patients with Stage $D_1$ prostatic
     adenocarcinoma. J. Urol. 125:817, 1981.

CHAPTER 5

MANAGEMENT OF ADVANCED PROSTATE CANCER

Marc B. Garnick

I.  SUMMARY OF VETERAN'S ADMINISTRATION COOPERATIVE UROLOGIC
    RESEARCH GROUP (VACURG) STUDIES

    A.  Entrance criteria for all VACURG studies
        1.  only newly diagnosed patients entered
        2.  all cases confirmed by reference pathologist
        3.  all acid phosphatase determinations centralized
        4.  all studies randomized prospectively

    B.  Summary of Study Designs (see Table 5-1.)

    C.  Ongoing Results and Conclusions
        1.  Study 1
            a.  5 mg DES reduced number of cancer deaths and
                retarded progression of disease; however, an
                excessive number of cardiovascular deaths
                occurred, especially in Stage III patients.
            b.  For Stage III patients randomized to placebo,
                less than 1/3 of patients died of prostate
                cancer.
            c.  Orchiectomy was not superior to 5 mg DES, and
                combination of the two was no better than
                either alone.
            d.  Patients whose initial therapy was placebo
                were:
                - more likely to have therapies changed
                - more likely to benefit from such change
                1) Estrogen, when used later in disease, was
                   not associated with increased
                   cardiovascular complications.

31

Table 5-1. Treatments studied and number of patients in stages
III and IV in the three major VACURG studies. Reproduced with
permission of the Publisher, Almquist and Wiskell Interna-
tional, Reference 8).

|                     | Number of patients |          |
|---------------------|----------|----------|
| Treatments[d]       | Stage III | Stage IV |
| *Study 1*[a]        |          |          |
| Placebo             | 261      | 223      |
| DES (5.0)           | 264      | 211      |
| Orch + Placebo      | 266      | 203      |
| Orch + DES (5.0)    | 258      | 216      |
| *Study 2*[b]        |          |          |
| Placebo             | 75       | 53       |
| DES (0.2)           | 73       | 52       |
| DES (1.0)           | 73       | 55       |
| DES (5.0)           | 73       | 54       |
| *Study 3*[c]        |          |          |
| Premarin (2.5)      | 140      | 123      |
| Provera (30.0)      | 136      | 119      |
| Provera (30.0) +    |          |          |
|   DES (1.0) | 134    | 117      |
| DES (1.0)           | 135      | 119      |

[a] Patients admitted from March 1960 through March
1967
[b] Patients admitted from April 1967 through May 1969.
[c] Patients admitted from June 1969 through September
1975.
[d] Treatment abbreviations: DES=diethylstilbestrol;
Orch=bilateral orchiectomy; daily doses in milligrams are
given in parentheses.

2. Study 2
   a. 5 mg DES confirmed to be hazardous, necessi-
      tating discontinuation of trial.
   b. 1 mg DES was as effective as 5 mg DES in
      retarding prostate cancer growth but did not
      increase cardiovascular mortality (endpoint
      used: rise in acid phosphatase, appearance of
      bony mets).
   c. 5 mg DES slightly better than 1 mg DES in
      decreasing size of primary lesion, decreasing
      plasma testosterone levels and decreasing
      acid phosphatase.
   d. 0.2 mg DES equaled placebo in overall effect.
   e. Choice of 1 mg DES recommended.
   f. 3 mg DES never tested by VACURG.

       g.  High risk group for cardiovascular complications was identified.

3. Study 3
    a.  No difference in any of the 4 treatments when overall survival used as endpoint.
    b.  No difference in survival curve when analyzed by cancer deaths only.


II. STAGE $D_2$ DISEASE – TREATMENT MODALITIES

The treatment program in patients with metastatic disease included hormonal therapy (previously referred to under the VA studies), cytotoxic chemotherapy, palliative radiation therapy for localized painful lesions and other investigational approaches. The various hormonal agents and the mechanism of action are listed below.

A. Hormonal Therapies (See also I. – VACURG Studies)
1. Stilphostral (diethylstilbestrol diphosphate) – for intravenous use, supposedly to allow increased concentration of DES to enter prostate cells.
2. Estradurin (polyestradiol phosphate) – sustained release form of estradiol for i.m. use.
3. Cyproterone acetate – predominantly progestational- –like agent that antagonizes androgen activity at level of androgen receptor.
4. Flutamide – non-steroidal antiandrogen that suppresses dihydrotestosterone receptor complex (in rats). Comparable to DES. "Estrogen" like side effects less frequent.
5. Tace (chlorotrianisene) – weakly estrogenic with ? mechanism of action similar to Flutamide.
6. Emcyt (estramustine phosphate) – estradiol 17-beta with mechlorethamine linked to the C3 of the steroid. Steroid moiety directs drug to susceptible cell. Phosphatases and hydrolases release alkylating agent intracellularly, thus avoiding systemic alkylating toxicity.
7. Prednimustine – prednisone linked with chlorambucil at C-21 (Leo-1031). Does cause myelosuppression.
8. Leuprolide – A gonadotropin releasing hormone analogue that decreases FSH, LH and effects significant responses in previously untreated

patients.  Much less toxic than DES.

B.  Chemotherapy for Advanced Prostate Cancer

Information concerning the efficacy of nonhormonal
chemotherapeutic agents for the treatment of prostatic cancer
has been limited.  Prior to the initiation of studies con-
ducted by the National Prostatic Cancer Group (NPCP) less than
10% of established anticancer agents had been adequately
tested in this disease.  The evaluation of objective responses
in prostate cancer is also very difficult, as many patients
have nonevaluable lesions.  The single agents which have been
reasonably well tested as well as others which are currently
undergoing evaluation and combination chemotherapeutic agents
are listed below.  Criteria established by the NPCP are
included.

1.  NPCP:  EVALUATION OF THERAPY CRITERIA

   a.  Partial Regression:
   .   50% reduction in measurable lesions
   .   Acid phosphatase return to normal
   .   Recalcification of "some" osteolytic lesions
       if present
   b.  Objectively Stable (all of following)
   .   Insufficient regression of primary indicator
       lesion
   .   less than 25% increase in any measurable
       lesion
   .   No significant weight loss (over 10%
       symptoms, or performance status (1 level)
   c.  Objective Progression (any of following)
   .   "Significant" deterioration in weight,
       symptoms, P.S.
   .   Appearance of new disease
   .   Increase by over 50% in pre-existing lesions
   .   Increase in acid/alkaline phosphatase not
       itself an indicator of progression.

## 2. SINGLE AGENT CHEMOTHERAPY

| Agent | N | Objective Response (ORR) (%) | ORR + Stable (%) |
|---|---|---|---|
| Cis-platinum (CDDP) | 70 | 21 | 36 |
| Adriamycin (ADR) | 83 | 23 | |
| Estramustine (EMP) | 319 | 18 | |
| Prednimustine (PRM) | 23 | 13 | |
| 5-FU | 48 | 10 | |
| Cyclophosphamide (CTX) | 120 | 14 | 37 |
| CCNU | 10 | 40 | |
| Melphalan | 15 | 7 | |
| Streptozotocin | 38 | – | 32 |
| DTIC | 23 | – | 39 |
| Methotrexate | 60 | – | 48 |

## 3. COMBINATION CHEMOTHERAPY TRIALS

| Agent | N | Objective Response (ORR) (%) | ORR + Stable (%) |
|---|---|---|---|
| CTX + 5 FU vs. | 18 | 11 | -- |
| ADR | 19 | 26 | -- |
| CTX + ADR | 35 | 26 | 7-69 |
| CTX + ADR + 5 FU vs. | 12 | -- | 50 |
| CTX | 15 | -- | 53 |
| CTX + ADR + BCNU | 22 | 32 | -- |
| CTX + ADR + MTX | 12 | -- | 75 |
| CDDP + ADR | 17 | 53 | -- |
| 5-FU + EMP | 25 | 32 | -- |
| 5-FU + MTX +VCR + Melphalan + pred-nisone | 25 | 24 | -- |
| EMP + PRM | 21 | 24 | -- |
| ADR + 5-FU + Mito C | 42 | 50 | -- |
| ADR + CTX + MTX | 12 | -- | 75 |
| ADR + CTX + CDDP | 16 | -- | 63 |

4.  RANDOMIZED TRIALS*:  SINGLE AGENTS vs.
    COMBINATION CHEMOTHERAPY

Single Agents    vs.   Combinations
5-FU                   5-FU + CTX + ADR
CTX                    CTX + ADR + 5-FU
Prednimustine (P)      (P) + Estramustine
                       phosphate(EMP)
CTX                    CTX + MTX + 5-FU
Vincristine (V)        V + EMP
EMP

---

*No difference noted between single agent vs. combination
in any of the trials.

III. ADJUVANT CHEMOTHERAPY FOR STAGE $D_1$

A series (not prospective) of 37 patients with Stage $D_1$
prostate cancer has evaluated the role of adjuvant chemotherapy.  Chemotherapy included cyclophosphamide (750 mg/$m_2$)
and adriamycin (50 mg/$m_2$) to a total adriamycin dose of 250
mg/$m_2$.  This data is summarized below.

|          | N  | N Progressing (%) | Time to Progression (mos.) |
|----------|----|-------------------|----------------------------|
| Treated  | 12 | 4 (33%)           | 15                         |
| Control  | 25 | 12 (48%)          | 11.6                       |

Although not statistically significant, these data emphasize
some possible use for adjuvant chemotherapy in high-risk
patients.  Recent follow-up suggests that overall survivorship
is not different between the groups.

IV.  CONCLUSIONS

.   Active agents include cyclophosphamide,
    5-fluorouracil, adriamycin, CDDP, estrogen
    preparations, Leuprolide.
.   Combination chemotherapy has not proven to be
    superior to single agents.
.   Pain relief and palliation may be achieved with
    chemotherapy.

- Improvement of survival not conclusively shown for chemotherapy.
- Entry of patients into clinical trials is encouraged to identify new, active agents.

SELECTED REFERENCES

VACURG Studies

1. Bailer, J.C., III, Byar, D.P. and VACURG:  Estrogen treatment for cancer of the prostate.  Cancer, 26:257, 1970.

2. Blackard, C.E.: The VACURG studies of carcinoma of the prostate: A review. Cancer Chemother Rep. 59:225, 1975.

3. Blackard CE, et al.:  Incidence of cardiovascular disease and death in patients receiving diethylstil- bestrol for carcinoma of the prostate.  Cancer 26:249, 1970.

4. Byar, D.P.:  The Veteran's Administration Cooperative Urological Research Group studies of cancer of the prostate.  Cancer 32:1126, 1973.

5. Byar, D.P.:  VACURG studies on prostatic cancer and its treatment.  In: Tannenbaum, M., ed. Urologic Pathology. The Prostate.  Philadelphia, Lea & Febiger, pp. 241-267, 1977.

6. Mellinger, G.T. and the Veterans' Administration Cooperative Urological Research Group:  Treatment and survival of patients with cancer of the prostate.  Surg. Gynec. Obstet. 124:1011, 1967.

7. The Veterans' Administration Cooperative Urological Research Group:  Factors in the prognosis of carcinoma of the prostate:  A cooperative study.  J. Urol. 100:59, 1968.

8. Byar, D.P.:  VACURG studies of conservative treatment. Scan. J. Urol. Nephrol. Suppl. 55:99, 1980.

CHEMOTHERAPY

9. Torti, F.M. and Carter, S.K.:  The chemotherapy of

prostatic adenocarcinoma.  Ann. Int. Med. 92:681, 1980.

10.  Schmidt, J.D.:  Chemotherapy of hormone resistant Stage D
     prostatic cancer.  J. Urol. 123:797, 1980.

11.  Garnick, M.B., Prout, G.R., Jr. and Canellos, G.P.:
     Cancer of the prostate.  In:  Holland, J.F., Frei, E.
     III, eds.  Cancer medicine.  Philadelphia: Lea and
     Febiger, second edition, pp. 1912-1934, 1982.

12.  Glode, L.M.: Leuprolide therapy of advanced prostate
     cancer.  Proc. Amer. Soc. Clin. Onc. 22:110, 1982.

13.  Cobau, C.D.:  Advances in management of carcinoma of the
     prostate. Amer. Soc. Clin. Onc. Educational Book, p. 48,
     1982.

14.  Loening, S.A., et al.:  Comparison of methotrexate,
     cis-platinum and estracyt in patients with advanced
     carcinoma of the prostate.  Proc Amer Urol Assoc, 1982
     Annual Meeting, Kansas City, MO; p. 152 (299),
     (Abstract).

15.  Soloway, M.S. et al.:  Comparison of estracyt,
     cis-platinum, and estracyt plus cis-platinum in patients
     with advanced, hormone resistant, previously irradiated
     carcinoma of prostate.  Proc Amer Urol Assoc. 1982 Annual
     Meeting, Kansas City, MO; p. 152 (300), (Abstract).

# SECTION II


## KIDNEY CANCER


New diagnostic methods and new therapeutic modalities are of the utmost import in renal cell carcinoma, an enigmatic tumor named "the internist's tumor" because of its bewildering array of clinical features. In this section, newer radio-graphic methods of diagnosis and staging are integrated into a systematic approach taking into consideration advances in radiologic imaging as well as the constraints of cost effect-iveness. Techniques of surgical management, including the individual patient with vena caval thrombus or with a solitary kidney, are considered in detail. The difficulties in selec-tion of treatment modalities for patients with advanced renal cell carcinoma have been updated, including consideration of immunotherapy. The evolution of treatment for Wilm's tumor, detailed by a surgeon, a radiotherapist, and a pediatric oncologist, represents a triumph of multimodality therapy that could serve as a template for the design of future trials.

CHAPTER 6

RENAL CELL CARCINOMA – DIAGNOSTIC WORKUP AND NATURAL HISTORY

Marc B. Garnick

I. EPIDEMIOLOGY AND ETIOLOGY

1.  The most common primary malignancy arising from the kidney in adults is renal cell carcinoma (RCC, renal adenocarcinoma), accounting for 2-3% of all cancer. In 1982, approximately 8,000 deaths due to renal cancer were documented (2.3% of male cancer deaths and 1.6% of female cancer deaths). The incidence of the disease is 7.5/100,000 population and is twice as common in males; Scandinavians and North Americans have the highest incidence; Asians and African, the lowest.

2.  The average age at presentation is between 55-60 years old.

3.  A moderate association between tobacco use and incidence of RCC has been found. A variety of chemical and biological agents have produced renal tumors in animals and include lead phosphate, dimethylnitrosamine, prolonged estrogen administration to male hamsters, aflatoxin ($B_1$), and viruses in leopard frogs. There is no conclusive evidence that any of these agents is causative in man, although some preliminary work indicates a potentially higher risk in cadmium workers who smoke.

4.  Hippel-Lindau disease, an autosomal dominant disease, is associated with retinal angiomas, hemangioblastomas of the CNS and may be associated with RCC, some of which are multiple.

5.  The drug streptozotocin can induce renal cancers in laboratory animals.

41

6.   Recently a 3-8 chromosomal translocation has been
     described in association with familial renal cancer.


II.  PATHOLOGY

1.   Renal adenocarinoma is the predominant type and is
     usually subclassified into clear cell, granular, and
     spindle tumors.  The term "hypernephroma" should be
     abandoned; the cell of origin is probably from
     tubular epithelium.
2.   There is some evidence that renal adenomas may be a
     precursor to the subsequent development of RCC in
     that some malignancies may evolve through a stage of
     adenomatous hyperplasia.


III. CLINICAL PRESENTATION

1.   RCC is extremely difficult to diagnose early in its
     course as there are few characteristic features.  The
     earlier complaints are usually weakness, weight loss,
     and anemia and occur in 1/3 of patients.  The diag-
     nostic triad of hematuria, flank pain, and mass
     occurs in only 10-12% and usually signifies metasta-
     tic disease in 50% of patients who present in this
     manner.  Overall, 1/3 of patients will have
     metastatic disease at presentation.

| A. LOCAL EFFECTS OF RCC | INCIDENCE(%) |
|---|---|
| i. Hematuria (usually painless, total) | 40 |
| ii. Flank pain | 50 |
| iii. Renal mass | 30 |
| iv. Acute varicocele | 3 |
| v. A-V fistulae(may be associated with high output CHF) | rare |
| vi. Hypertension | common (equal to incidence for age group) |

B.    SYSTEMIC AND PARANEOPLASTIC EFFECTS OF RCC

|  |  | INCIDENCE(%) |
|---|---|---|
| i. | Malaise, weight loss, anemia | 33 |
| ii. | Fever (in assoc. c̄ other abnormalities) | 17 |
|  | a. Fever(as sole presenting features | 2 |
| iii. | Abnormal, nonmetastatic liver chemistries | 0-12 |
| iv. | Amyloidosis | 4 |
| v. | Neuromyopathy | 4 |
| vi. | Erythrocytosis ($2^o$) | 4 |
| vii. | Elevated ESR | 50 |
| viii. | Hypertension (renin mediated) | (CR)* |
| ix. | Hypercalcemia (PTH mediated) | (CR)* |
| x. | Enteropathy ($2^o$ to glucagon) | (CR)* |
| xi. | Others: Prolactin, prostaglandins corticosteroids, ACTH | (CR)* |

*Case Reports

C.       OTHER UNUSUAL PRESENTATIONS

    i. 11 year history of abdominal mass with history of polycystic kidney.
   ii. Chest pain, dyspnea, $2^o$ to RCC blocking IVC.
  iii. Calcific renal mass in patient with 12 year history of breast cancer.
   iv. Immune complex glomerulonephritis.
    v. Renal hemorrhage following anticoagulation for an MI.

Renal cell carcinoma can masquerade in many guises.  The nonspecificity of the symptoms and presenting manifestations should always bring the diagnosis of RCC to mind.


IV.  DIAGNOSTIC EVALUATION

   1. Radiographic tests:

    A.  Flat plate of abdomen: Tumor may contain calcifications (nonspecific).

B.  IVP: 90% of RCC will demonstrate a space-
    occupying lesion. Nephrotomography is extremely
    useful in identifying lucent (cystic) and solid
    defects.

C.  Ultrasonography:  can help delineate solid from
    cystic lesions.

D.  Selective renal arteriography: usually performed
    via the transfemoral route may demonstrate
    typical neovascularity and pooling and tumor
    blush and may be accentuated with epinephrine
    injection.  Renal arteriography has added
    measurably in differentiating cysts from tumors.
    Diagnostic problems which are occasionally
    difficult to distinguish include
    xanthogranulomatous pyelonephritis, hamartoma and
    metastatic lesions.

E.  Abdominal CT scan: promising and may now be
    considered diagnostic procedure of choice.

F.  Cyst puncture.

If renal cell carcinoma is suspected, a suggested flow
diagram (Figure 6-1) is seen below.

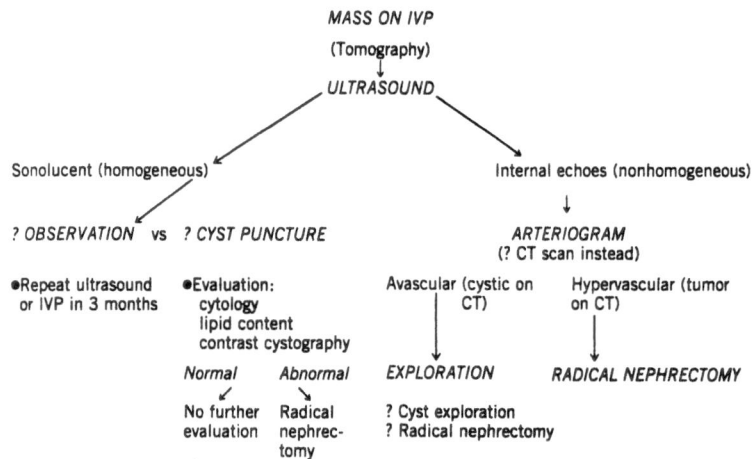

Figure 6-1.  Radiographic evaluation and treatment of
suspected renal mass. (Reproduced with permission, Lea and
Febiger, Philadephia, Ref. 29).

2.  Steps in metastatic workup:  Metastatic disease is
    present in approximately 1/3 of patients upon initial
    presentation.  The most distant sites of involvement
    are as follows:

|  | INCIDENCE(%) |
|---|---|
| Lung (commonly endobronchial) | 50 |
| Bone (osteolytic) | 32 |
| Brain and thyroid | 25 |
| Local invasion to adrenal, colon, spleen, diaphragm | 9 each |
| Liver | 33 |

3.  If renal cell carcinoma is suspected, assess staging
    preoperatively with studies directed at documenting
    metastatic disease.


V.  SURGICAL AND PATHOLOGICAL STAGING

1.  Stage I:    Tumor confined to renal parenchyma.
    Stage II:   Perinephric fat involvement but confined
                to Gerota's fascia.
    Stage III:  Involvement of regional lymph nodes and/or
                renal vein or inferior vena cava.
    Stage IV:   Involvement of adjacent organs (usually
                not adrenal) and distant metastatic
                disease.

2.  Histologic Grading:

                              Prognosis

    A. Cell Type
        i. Clear              1. Pure clear cell
       ii. Granular              tumor may have
      iii. Spindle               better prognosis.
                              2. Spindle cell worse.

    B. Organization           1. Alveolar, no influ-
        i. Tubular               ence on survival;
       ii. Papillary             however, Stage I
      iii. Alveolar              papillary may have
       iv. Sheet                 survival advantage.

    C. Nuclear                1. Nuclear morphology
       Structure              (if correlated with stage)
                              may be predictive.

3.  Survival by Stage:

| Stage | N | 5-year | N | 10-year |
|-------|----|--------|----|---------|
| I | 32 | 66% | 15 | 60% |
| II | 15 | 64% | 6 | 67% |
| III | 24 | 42% | 13 | 38% |
| IV | 9 | 11% | 3 | 0% |

Several others series in patients presenting with metastatic disease indicate a 25% one-year survival and less than 5% at three years.

4.  Prognostic Factors:
    1.  Size of lesion: lesions less than 3 cm rarely associated with metastases, while incidence of metastases increases if the primary lesion is greater than 6 cm.
    2.  Multifocality: worse prognosis if tumors are multicentric.
    3.  Stage of disease: higher stage, lower survival.
    4.  Type of nephrectomy: controversial, but most perform radical nephrectomy.
    5.  Renal vein involvement: majority of studies indicate poorer survival if present. (See also chapter 7).
    6.  Adjuvant radiation therapy: probably no benefit in survival, but preoperative radiation therapy may decrease local recurrence rate and diminish size of initial lesions.

VI.  MANAGEMENT OF DISSEMINATED DISEASE

   A. 1.  Carefully selected patients may benefit if solitary metastases are surgically removed.
        i.   Long time interval between nephrectomy and appearance of metastases is a subgroup which favors a good result.
        ii.  The presence of necrosis in the histological specimen has been associated with a good result from surgical removal of metastases.
      2.  In the presence of metastatic disease, nephrectomy may be justified if the patient is experiencing local pain or bleeding.

3. Spontaneous regression of metastases is extremely rare but has been reported in approximately 60 cases and rarely followed nephrectomy.
4. Adjunctive nephrectomy in patients with osseous disease only has been associated with some prolongation of survival.

B. CHEMOTHERAPY AND HORMONAL THERAPY IN ADVANCED RENAL CELL CARCINOMA (See Also Chapter 9).

| Agent | N | CR(%) | CR + PR(%) |
|-------|---|-------|------------|
| Progestins | 61 | 0 | 11 |
| Androgens | 37 | 0 | 0 |
| CCNU | 79 | 0 | 10 |
| MeCCNU | 45 | 0 | 4 |
| Cyclophosphamide | 22 | 0 | 4 |
| Hydroxyurea | 25 | 0 | 28 |
| 5-Fluorouracil | 40 | 0 | 8 |
| Vinblastine (VBL) | 44 | 4 | 9 |
| VBL + CCNU | 29 | 7 | 24 |
| VBL + Progestin | 38 | 0 | 8 |
| MeCCNU + Progestin | 38 | 2 | 10 |
| ADR + VCR + Progestin + BCG | 31 | 0 | 33 |

VII. METASTATIC LESIONS TO KIDNEY

1. Most Common:  lung.
2. Lymphoma involvement is extremely common but rarely causes functional abnormalities.

SELECTED REFERENCES

1. Richie, J.P. and Skinner, D.G.: Renal neoplasia. In: Brenner, B. and Rector, E., eds.: The Kidney. Philadelphia: W.B. Saunders, second edition, p. 2109, 1981.

2. Kantor, A.F.: Current concepts in the epidemiology and etiology of primary renal cell carcinoma.  J. Urol 117:415, 1977.

3.  Kantor, A.L.F., et al.: Epidemiology of renal cell
    carcinoma in Connecticut. J.N.C.I. 57:495, 1976.

4.  Wynder, E.L., Mabuschi, K. and Whitmore, W.F., Jr.:
    Epidemiology of adenocarcinoma of the kidney. J.N.C.I.
    53:1619, 1974.

5.  Holland, J.M.: Natural history and staging of renal cell
    carcinoma.  CA-A Journal for Clinicians 25:121, 1975.

6.  Waters, W.B. and Richie, J.P.: Aggressive surgical
    approach to renal cell carcinoma: Review of 130 cases. J.
    Urol. 122:306, 1979.

7.  Kolonel, L.N.: Association of cadmium with renal cancer.
    Cancer 37:1782, 1976.

8.  Cronin, R.E., et al.: Renal cell carcinoma: Unusual
    systemic manifestations. Medicine 55:291, 1976.

9.  Lebel, M., et al.: Adenocarcinoma of the kidney and
    hypertension: Report of 2 cases with special emphasis on
    renin. J. Urol. 118:923, 1977

10. Boxer, R.J., et al.: Nonmetastatic hepatic dysfunction
    associated with renal carcinoma. J. Urol. 119:468, 1978.

11. Karcioglu, Z.A., et al.: Trace element concentrations in
    renal cell carcinoma. Cancer 42:1330, 1978.

12. McPhedran, P., et al.: Alpha-2 globulin "spike" in renal
    carcinoma. Ann. Int. Med. 76:439, 1972.

13. Cummings, K.B. and Robertson, R.P.: Prostaglandin:
    Increased production by renal cell carcinoma. J. Urol.
    118:720, 1977.

14. Schefft, P., et al.: Surgery for renal cell carcinoma
    extending into the inferior vena cava. J. Urol. 120:28,
    1978.

15. Viets, D.H., Vaughan, D., Jr. and Howards, S.S.:
    Experience gained from the management of 9 cases of
    bilateral renal cell carcinoma. J. Urol. 118:937, 1977.

16. Montie, J.E., et al.: The role of adjunctive nephrectomy in patients with metastatic renal cell carcinoma. J. Urol. 117:272, 1977.

17. Concolino, G., et al.: Human renal cell carcinoma as a hormone-dependent tumor. Canc. Res. 38:4340, 1978.

18. Lokich, J.J. and Harrison, J.H.: Renal cell carcinoma: Natural history and chemotherapeutic experience. J. Urol. 114:371, 1975.

19. Katakkar, S.B. and Franks, C.R.: Chemo-hormonal therapy for metastatic renal cell carcinoma with adriamycin, hydroxyurea, vinblastine and medroxyprogesterone acetate. Cancer Treat. Rep. 62:1379, 1978.

20. Mittelman, A., Albert. D.J. and Murphy, G.P.: Lomustine treatment of metastatic renal cell carcinoma, JAMA 225:32, 1973.

21. Kiruluta, G., Morales, A. and Lott., S.: Response of renal adenocarcinoma to cyclophosphamide. Urol. 6:557, 1975.

22. Alberto, O. and Senn, H.J.: Hormonal therapy of renal carcinoma alone and in association with cytostatic drugs. Cancer 33:1226, 1974.

23. Hahn, R.G., et al.: Phase II study of vinblastine, methyl-CCNU,and medroxyprogesterone in advanced renal cell cancer. Cancer Treat. Rep. 62:1093, 1978.

24. Talley, R.: Chemotherapy of adenocarcinoma of the kidney. Cancer 32:1062, 1973.

25. Carter, S.K. and Wasserman, T.H.: The chemotherapy of urologic cancer. Cancer 36:729, 1975.

26. Rubenstein, M.A., Walz, B.J. and Bucy, J.G.: Transitional cell carcinoma of the kidney: 25 year experience. J. Urol. 119:594, 1978.

27. Richmond, J., et al: Renal lesions associated with malignant lymphomas. Amer. J. Med. 32:184, 1962.

28. Patel, N.P. and Lavengood, R.W.: Renal cell carcinoma:
    Natural history and results of treatment. J. Urol.
    119:722, 1978.

29. Richie, J.P. and Garnick, M.B.: Primary renal and ureteral
    cancer.  In: Rieselbach, R.E. and Garnick, M.B., eds.:
    Cancer and The Kidney, Philadelphia: Lea and Febiger,
    p. 662, 1982.

CHAPTER 7

SURGICAL MANAGEMENT OF RENAL CELL CARCINOMA


Jerome P. Richie


The best treatment to date for renal cell carcinoma is
total surgical extirpation.  Prior to the 1960s, removal of
the kidney for renal cell carcinoma was accomplished by simple
nephrectomy.  Robson, in 1963, described the now standard
approach of radical nephrectomy.  Radical nephrectomy is
accomplished by early ligation of the renal artery and renal
vein, en bloc removal of the kidney with surrounding Gerota's
fascia, and removal of the regional lymph nodes.  With
Robson's report of an improved 5 year survival rate of 66%
compared to previous cumulative surgical survival rates of 48%
for simple nephrectomy, radical nephrectomy has become the
procedure of choice.
    Various surgical approaches are available for the effec-
tive performance of this procedure.  The thoraco-abdominal
approach, described by Chute and associates, offers the distinct advantage of palpation of the ipsilateral lung cavity
and mediastinum and the ability to resect solitary pulmonary
metastases.  Alternative approaches include an extrapleural
supracostal incision or an anterior transabdominal incision.
Regardless of which approach is utilized, the principle of
early ligation of the vascular pedicle is important to prevent
dissemination of tumor at the time of operation.


REGIONAL LYMPHADENECTOMY

    Involvement of the regional lymphatics and periaortic
lymph nodes has been noted in almost 25% of patients with
renal cell carcinoma.  Hence, the rationale exists for
regional lymphadenectomy to be performed in conjunction

51

with radical nephrectomy.  The major value of identification
of regional lymph node involvement would seem to be its prognostic import, although an occasional patient with one or two
positive nodes has been shown to be a long-term survivor.
Nevertheless, because the five-year survival in patients with
regional nodal involvement is substantially less than that in
patients with stages I and II tumors, this factor may be
important in the design of trials for adjuvant therapy.
Regional lymphadenectomy adds little in terms of operative
time or risk and should be included in conjunction with
radical nephrectomy.

RENAL VEIN AND/OR INFERIOR VENA CAVAL INVOLVEMENT

     Approximately 5% of patients with renal cell carcinoma
have inferior vena caval involvement.  Tumor invasion of the
renal vein and inferior vena cava usually occurs as a well-
vascularized thrombus covered with its own intimal surface,
and this has important bearing for surgical planning and
approach.  In such instances, and in the absence of demon-
strable metastases, radical nephrectomy is performed with
early ligation of the renal artery, but no manipulation of the
renal vein.  Vascular control of the inferior vena cava is
obtained above and below the tumor thrombus, and radical
nephrectomy is carried out in standard fashion.  Once the
tumor has been mobilized completely, a venacavotomy can be
performed with extraction of tumor thrombus (occassionally up
to the right atrium if necessary with cardiopulmonary bypass)
and closure of the vena cava.  An occasional tumor may actually invade the inferior vena cava, necessitating inferior
vena caval resection as described by McCullough and Gittes.
However, survival in those patients with actual invasion of
the inferior vena caval wall is poor in the absence of effective adjuvant therapy.

PROGNOSIS

     Five-year survival after radical nephrectomy for stage I
renal cell carcinoma ranges from 60 to 75%, and patients with
stage II lesions have a survival from 47 to 65%.  Patients
with renal vein or inferior vena caval involvement have a
survival of 25 to 50%, and patients with regional lymph node
involvement or extracapsular extension have a survival of 12
to 25%.

In the patient with effective surgical removal of renal vein or inferior vena caval thrombus, five-year survivals of 25 to 50% have been reported. Based upon our review of patients at the Brigham and Women's Hospital, renal vein involvement alone does not carry a more ominous prognosis. Thus, we feel that renal vein involvement should be a subclassification of stage II rather than stage III. Inferior vena caval involvement alone carries a five-year survival of approximately 25%, certainly better than that seen in patients with positive nodal involvement.


TUMORS IN THE SOLITARY KIDNEY OR BILATERAL SIMULTANEOUS TUMORS

Over 90 cases of renal cell carcinoma arising in a solitary kidney have been reported, and the subject has been extensively reviewed by Wickham. Until recently, the only techniques available for management of the tumor in the solitary kidney included partial nephrectomy (preferably for polar lesions) or radical nephrectomy and institution of dialysis with possible later renal transplantation. Recent advances in transplantation and renal preservation, as well as more aggressive surgical techniques, have allowed management of larger or centrally located tumors by two additional methods: in vivo partial nephrectomy with local hypothermia or ex vivo "workbench" surgery with subsequent autotransplantation. The majority of tumors in solitary kidneys can be adequately managed by in vivo partial nephrectomy techniques, but occasionally workbench surgery with autotransplantation is necessary.

Wickham concluded that if the contralateral kidney had been removed for previous renal cell carcinoma, survival was not as good as if the contralateral kidney had been removed for benign disease or was congenitally absent. However, a review of his own data showed that within each category survival rates were improved in patients who underwent partial nephrectomy as primary therapy rather than no treatment. Novick and associates, in a review of 64 patients reported in the literature with tumor in a solitary kidney, found no difference in overall survival whether the contralateral kidney was removed for carcinoma or not. The results of intensive therapy by partial nephrectomy in a patient with a solitary kidney support the contention that a potentially resectable tumor can be excised whenever permitted by the patient's medical condition and physical status.

Patients with bilateral synchronous renal cell carci-

noma often have evidence of other disseminated disease. Few
such patients survive two years even with radical nephrectomy
and partial nephrectomy.  Nonetheless, if distant metastases
have been excluded, the most reasonable approach would be to
treat the contralateral renal involvement as a solitary metastasis and to excise by partial nephrectomy when feasible.
Simultaneous surgical management can be offered through an
anterior abdominal (Chevron) incision.

The option of complete radical nephrectomy and chronic
hemodialysis is one that can be considered in certain
patients.  The risks of chronic hemodialysis are considerable,
and transplantation with immunosuppression raises the unknown
risk of tumor recurrence.  However, satisfactory long-term
results have been reported by Calne.


PREOPERATIVE ARTERIAL EMBOLIZATION

Percutaneous transaortic embolization of the main renal
artery has been advocated as a procedure to diminish blood
loss, especially in patients with large or locally invasive
tumors.  This approach helps simplify the radical nephrectomy
by allowing ligation of the main renal vein initially rather
than dissection more posteriorly to ligate the renal artery
first.  Several investigators have hypothesized that infarction of the tumor enhances the immune response.  The procedure
of arterial embolization has been associated with complications, including potential distal emboli, pain, fever, and
generalized malaise.  Because renal cell carcinomas parasitize
other vessels, infarction of the tumors is seldom complete.
Furthermore, numerous venous collaterals must still be dealt
with intraoperatively, and blood loss has been reduced only
minimally.  In general, angioinfarction should be reserved for
the very selected patient and has not seemed to expedite
radical nephrectomy in the majority.


SUGGESTED REFERENCES

1.  Freed, S.Z. and Gliedman, M.L.: The removal of renal
    carcinoma thrombus extending into the right atrium. J.
    Urol. 113:163, 1975.

2.  Kearney, G.P. et al: Results of inferior vena cava
    resection for renal cell carcinoma.  J. Urol. 125:769,
    1981.

3.  McCullough, D.L. and Gittes, R.F.: Ligation of the renal
    vein in the solitary kidney: Effects on renal function. J.
    Urol. 113:295, 1975.

4.  Novick, A.C., et al.: Partial nephrectomy in the treatment
    of renal adenocarcinoma. J. Urol. 118:932, 1977.

5.  Robson, C.J.: Radical nephrectomy for renal cell
    carcinoma. J. Urol. 89:37, 1963.

6.  Schefft, P., et al.: Surgery for renal cell carcinoma
    extending into inferior vena cava. J. Urol. 120:28, 1978.

7.  Skinner, D.G. and deKernion, J.B.: Clinical manifestations
    and treatment of renal parenchymal tumors.  In Skinner,
    D.G. and deKernion, J.B., eds: Genitourinary Cancer.
    Philadelphia:  W.B. Saunders Co., p. 107, 1978.

8.  Waters, W.B. and Richie, J.P.: Aggressive surgical
    approach to renal cell carcinoma: Review of 130 cases. J.
    Urol. 122:306, 1979.

9.  Wickham, J.E.A.: Conservative renal surgery for
    adenocarcinoma. The place of bench surgery. Br. J. Urol.
    47:25, 1975.

10. Richie, J.P. and Garnick, M.B.  Primary renal and ureteral
    cancer. In: Rieselbach, R.E. and Garnick, M.B., eds.:
    Cancer and the Kidney.  Philadephia: Lea and Febiger,
    p. 662, 1982.

CHAPTER 8

THE ROLE OF RADIATION THERAPY IN RENAL CARCINOMA

Leslie Botnick

I.  Adenocarcinomas of the renal parenchyma have a radio-
    sensitivity that is similar to other glandular tumors.

    A.  Moderate doses of radiation (3000-4000 rad) cause
        tumor regression.
    B.  However, inability to give curative doses of
        radiation (greater than 6000 rad) to the tumorous
        region without excessive normal tissue toxicity
        makes radiation unlikely to be useful as primary
        modality.

II. Whether radiation (dose range 3000-4000 rad) preopera-
    tively can facilitate surgical removal of the tumor and
    prolong patient survival is controversial.

    A.  Preoperative radiation increases the resectability
        rate and improves local control.
    B.  Retrospective studies suggest improved resect-
        ability and long term survival.
    C.  Some prospective studies confirm the increased
        resectability rate with preoperative radiation for
        advanced disease but not improved survival.  Others
        cannot confirm either observation.

III. Since it is unlikely for radiation to be of benefit for
     all types of renal cancer, can one select a group of
     patients who have a stage of disease that can be
     treated postoperatively after tumor removal and

surgical staging?

A.  Some studies retrospectively note improved survival
    and local control in patients treated with extra-
    renal extension, renal pelvis involvement, or lymph
    node involvement.
B.  Others cannot show any pathologic or staging
    criteria which demonstrates a beneficial effect of
    radiation.


IV.  One cannot conclusively demonstrate a benefit for
     either pre-or post-operative radiation for all patients
     regardless of stage.

A.  However, with CT scan one may be able to select
    inoperable or borderline operable patients for
    preoperative treatment and hopefully improve
    resectability.
B.  Intraoperative radiation may be useful as a boost
    to areas where gross residual disease is left
    behind.  Thereafter external radiation to tolerance
    doses can be used (4000-5000 rad) to possible areas
    of microscopic disease in selected patients.

SUGGESTED REFERENCES

1.  Bratherton: The place of radiotherapy in the treatment of
    hypernephroma. Br. J. Radiol. 34:141, 1964.

2.  Finney, R: The value of radiotherapy in the treatment of
    hypernephroma--A clinical trial. Br. J. Urol. 45:258,
    1973.

3.  Flocks, R.T.T. and Kadesky, M.C.: Malignant neoplasms of
    the kidney: analysis of 353 patients followed five years
    or more. J. Urol. 79:196, 1958.

4.  Juusela, H., Malmia, K., Alfthan, O. and OraVisto K.J.:
    Preoperative irradiation in the treatment of renal
    adenocarcinoma. Scand. J. Urol. Nephrol. 11:277, 1977.

5.  Peeling, W.B., Mantell, B.S. and Shepheard, B.G.F.:
    Postoperative irradiation in the treatment of renal cell
    carcinoma. Br. J. Urol. 41:23, 1969.

6.  Riches, E.W., Griffiths, I.H. and Thackray, A.C.: New
    growths of the kidney and ureter. Br. J. Urol. 23:297,
    1951.

7.  Rost, A. and Brasig, W: Preoperative irradiation of renal
    cell carcinoma. Urol. 10:414, 1977.

8.  Waters, C.A.: Preoperative irradiation of cortical renal
    tumors. Am.J. Roentgenol. Radium Ther. 33:149, 1935.

9.  Van der Werf-Messing, B.: Cancer of the kidney. Cancer
    32:1056, 1973.

CHAPTER 9

MANAGEMENT OF ISOLATED METASTASES AND ADVANCED RENAL CARCINOMA

George P. Canellos


I. SURGERY

A. Palliative Nephrectomy

1. Acceptable for relief of severe local symptoms
such as pain, hemorrhage, and possible endocrino-
pathic features refractory to symptomatic
treatment.
2. Unacceptable in patients without local symptoms
but with metastatic disease.
3. Induction of spontaneous regression by nephrectomy
a. Overall incidence of this event 4/571
neph-rectomies (0.8%).
b. surgical mortality - 2-15%
c. cumulative survival of palliative
nephrectomy patients unchanged from that
of a series of metastatic renal cell
cancer patients.
4. Indications for palliative nephrectomy include:
a. patients with solitary metastases
(excised)
b. patients who responded to some form of
systemic therapy.
5. Survival. Middleton reported on 59 patients with
excision of solitary metastases and palliative
nephrectomy: 45%-3yr and 34%-5yr. survival.
Katzenstein et al. reported on 12 patients with
excision of pulmonary metastases and nephrectomy.
Two of 3 pts with bilateral metastases died after

61

more than 12 mos. Three of 8 pts with unilateral
metastases died 12, 15, 29 mos. Three pts. alive
without disease, 1 with disease, 1 lost to follow-up.

B.  Solitary Metastases

Metastatic disease at diagnosis occurs in 20-30% of
patients.  In the vast majority, multiple metastases
occur.  Middleton et al. reported that 141/503 pts. presented with multiple metastases and 81/503 presented with
solitary metastases.
Skinner et al. reported that 62/329 (19%) had distant
metastasis at presentation.

1.  Excisions of metastases from renal cancer patients
    involve primarily pulmonary wedge resection
    a.  brain, opposite kidney, thyroid, bone and retro-
        peritoneum also reported.
    b.  long survival after excision of solitary or
        multiple metastases is anecdotal.
    c.  the majority of long survivors had a solitary
        metastasis excised many years after primary
        nephrectomy.
2.  Excision of Pulmonary Metastases
    a.  Favorable prognostic features:
        i. Negative tracheobronchial nodes
        ii. Necrosis
    b.  Features without Prognostic Significance:
        i. Size of metastases
        ii. Microscopic lung metastases
    c.  Negative prognostic features include:
        i. Extension to pleura, chest wall, diaphragm or
           mediastinum.
        ii. Multiple metastases seen on radiographs
3.  Presenting symptoms-cough, dyspnea, hemoptysis- often
    asymptomatic
4.  Wedge resection in 75% of cases with lobectomy in 20%.
5.  Survival following resection

|                        | # of Patients | 5 yr Survival |
|------------------------|---------------|---------------|
| Morrow et al.          | 23            | 24%           |
| Skinner et al.         | 24            | 33 1/3%       |
| Katzenstein et al.     | 44            | 30%           |

7.  Advanced renal cell cancer has no standard therapy
    and thus, experimental treatments with new drugs,
    such as interferon, are appropriate.

SELECTED REFERENCES

SURGERY (Palliative Nephrectomy)

1.  DeKernion, J.B. and Berry, D.:  The diagnosis and
    treatment of renal cell cell carcinoma.  Cancer 45:1947,
    1980.

2.  Katzenstein, A.L., et al.:  Pulmonary resection for
    metastatic renal adenocarcinoma.  Cancer 41:712, 1978.

3.  Middleton, R.G.,:  The value of surgery in metastatic
    renal cell carcinoma.  In: King, J.S., ed.: Renal
    Neoplasia, Boston: Little, Brown and Company, p. 483,
    1964.


SURGERY (Solitary Metastases)

4.  Middleton, R.G.:  Surgery for metastatic renal cell
    carcinoma.  J. Urol. 97:973, 1967.

5.  Morrow, C.E., Vassilopoulos, P.P. and Grage, T.B.:
    Surgical resection for metastatic neoplasms of the lung.
    Cancer 45:2981, 1980.

6.  Skinner, D.G. et al.:  Diagnosis and management of renal
    cell carcinoma.  Cancer 28:1165, 1971.

RADIATION THERAPY

7.  Van der Werf-Messing, B.:  Carcinoma of the kidney.
    Cancer 32:1056, 1973.


ARTERIAL OCCLUSION

8.  Johnson, D.E., et al.:  Arterial occlusive techniques in
    the management of renal disease.  Weekly Urol. Update
    Ser. 1:1, 1978.

IMMUNOTHERAPY

9.  Cox, C.E., et al.:  Renal adenocarcinoma:  28 years
    review, with emphasis on rationale and feasibility of
    preoperative radiotherapy.  J. Urol. 104:53, 1970.

10. Humphrey, L.J., Murray, D.R. and Boehm, O.R.: Effective
    tumor vaccines in immunizing patients with cancer.  Surg.
    Gynecol. Obstet. 132:437, 1971.

11. Montie, J.E., Bukowsla, R.M. and Deodhar, S.D.:
    Immunotherapy of disseminated renal cell carcinoma with
    transfer factor.  J. Urol. 117:553, 1977.

12. Ramming, K.P. and deKernion, J.B.:  Immune RNA therapy for
    renal cell carcinoma.  Survival and immunologic monitor-
    ing.  Ann. Surg. 186:459, 1977.

13. Richie, J.P., et al.:  In vivo and in vitro effects of
    xenogeneic immune ribonucleic acid in patients with
    advanced renal cell carcinoma:  A phase I study.  J. Urol.
    126:24, 1981.

14. Skinner, D.G., et al.:  Advanced renal cell carcinoma:
    Treatment with xenogeneic immune ribonucleic acid  and
    appropriate surgical resection.  J. Urol. 115:246, 1976.


CHEMOTHERAPY

15. Katakkar, S.B. and Franks, C.R.:  Chemo-hormonal therapy
    for metastatic renal cell carcinoma with Adriamycin,
    hydroxyurea, vinblastine and medroxyprogesterone acetate.
    Cancer Treat. Rep. 62:1379, 1978.

16. Poster, D.S. et al.:  Current status of chemotherapy,
    hormonal therapy, and immunotherapy in the treatment of
    renal cell carcinoma.  Am. J. Clin. Oncol. 5:53, 1982.

17. Richards, F., II, et al.:  CCNU, Bleomycin, and
    Methylprednisolone with or without Adriamycin in renal
    cell carcinoma:  A randomized trial.  Cancer Treat. Rep.
    61:1591, 1977.

HORMONAL THERAPY

18. Bloom, H.J.G.:  Medroxyprogesterone acetate (Provera) in the treatment of metastatic renal cancer.  Brit. J. Cancer 25:250, 1971.

19. Concolino, G., et al.:  Human renal cell carcinoma as a hormone-dependent tumor.  Cancer Res. 38:4340, 1978.

CHAPTER 10

CANCERS OF THE RENAL PELVIS AND URETER


Marc B. Garnick and Jerome P. Richie



I.  DEMOGRAPHIC INFORMATION

    1. Renal pelvis and ureteral tumors constitute 5% of
       all kidney neoplasms:
       a. bladder: renal pelvis: ureter: 51:3:1.
       b. autopsy incidence 1/1000.

    2. Peak age incidence fifth to sixth decade.

    3. Male: Female: 2:1

    4. Ureteral tumors more commonly involve lower 1/3 of
       ureter


II. ETIOLOGIC FACTORS

    1. Workers in aniline dye, rubber, textile, and plastic
       industries have increased incidence of transitional
       cell cancer (TCC).

    2. Schistosomiasis, cigarette smoking, and exposure to
       viruses have been implicated in the genesis of
       urothelial neoplasms.

    3. Analgesic nephropathy and Balkan nephropathy have
       been strongly implicated in the development of renal
       pelvic cancer.

III.  PRESENTING SIGNS AND SYMPTOMS

    1. Hematuria: 75% will demonstrate this symptom during
       the disease course.

    2. Urinary frequency, malaise, weight loss, inanition,
       fever are not uncommon complaints.

    3. Urinary irritative symptoms more common in patients
       with ureteral tumors (50%) than those with renal
       pelvic tumors (10%).
       a. delay in diagnosis is common, with average
          duration lasting two months to two years.


IV.  PATHOLOGIC GRADING AND STAGING

    1. Histopathologic types
       a. TCC $\pm$ glandular or squamous differentiation: 90%
       b. squamous cell carcinoma (SCC): 8%
       c. adenocarcinoma: approximately 2%

    2. TCC
       a. Broders' classification generally employed
       b. Controversy does surround distinction between
          papilloma from low grade papillary carcinoma.
       c. Staging (ureteral tumors)
              Stage 0:   strictly limited to mucosa
              Stage A:   invasion of lamina propria
                         without muscular invasion
              Stage B:   confined to muscularis
              Stage C:   invasion of serosa
              Stage D:   distant metastases
       d. Staging (renal pelvic tumors)
              Similar to staging for bladder cancers.
       e. Both lymphatic and hematogenous metastases occur

    3. SCC
       a. Commonly associated with initiation of a renal
          pelvic calculus and pre-existing squamous
          metaplasia or leukoplakia.
       b. Most present with stage C or D disease.
       c. Hematuria occurs late; cytology not useful.
    4. Adenocarcinoma
       a. 60 cases reported; most with Stage D disease.

V.   DIAGNOSTIC TECHNIQUES

   1. <u>IVP</u>:  initial diagnostic procedure; tumors usually
      delineated as radiolucent filling defect.
      a. with far advanced disease, nonvisualization may
         occur in 6%, and hydronephrosis in 34%.
      b. filling defects usually further evaluated with
         retrograde pyelography.

   2. <u>Retrograde Pyelography</u>: should be utilized to obtain
      urinary washings, cytology and passage of ureteral
      brush.  May help delineate clot from tumor or tumor
      from radiolucent calculus (Bergman's sign).  This
      procedure also allows delineation of multiple
      filling defects in ureter not suspected on basis of
      IVP.

   3. Other radiographic studies:
      a. Antegrade pyelography may be useful in selected
         circumstances; arteriography usually is of little
         benefit.

   4. Cytology
      a. may be very useful in establishing the diagnosis
         of TCC.
      b. A positive cytology in filling defect in renal
         pelvis or ureter usually diagnostic of a TCC.

   5. Brush Biopsy
      a. may increase diagnostic accuracy in upper tract
         filling defects.


VI.   TREATMENT

   1. Radical operative therapy: nephrouretectomy plus
      cuff of bladder that includes ipsilateral ureteral
      orifice has been most recommended surgery.  This
      procedure allows accurate estimate of stage, and may
      help prevent subsequent ureteral stump recurrences.

   2. Conservative operative therapy: is indicated in
      patients with solitary kidney, decreased renal
      function, bilateral lesions, endemic Balkan
      nephropathy.

3. General philosophy: "The choice of treatment for patients with renal pelvic and ureteral tumors remains controversial. Patients with localized defects, presumably grade I and Stage A tumors, may well be treated by conservative means. In patients with more advanced tumors, however, the likelihood of ipsilateral ureteral recurrence, carcinoma-in-situ in the ipsilateral ureter, and the lack of effective ancillary therapies for patients with recurrences or distant metastases would seem to favor early and aggressive operative intervention. The low reported incidence of bilaterality (less than 5%) would also favor removing an ipsilateral system in order to prevent further tumor recurrences. Regardless of the form of therapy, however, one must remain congnizant of the possibility of other urothelial recurrences and evaluate the bladder at periodic intervals, as bladder cancers may be the first site of recurrence in a large proportion of patients." (21)

4. Radiation Therapy
   a. Role of radiation therapy not well defined; some investigators have advocated either preoperative or postoperative radiation therapy.
      Post operative XRT may be reasonable in patients with Stage B or C disease

5. Chemotherapy
   a. Various agents have been used. None can be considered as standard therapy. Role of superficial therapy with thiotepa and adriamycin still being investigated for low grade lesions.

SELECTED REFERENCES

1. Richie, J.P. and Garnick, M.B. Primary Renal and Ureter Cancer. In: Rieselbach R.E. and Garnick, M.B., ed.: Cancer and the Kidney, Philadelphia: Lea and Febiger, 1982, p. 662.

2. Davin, T., Cosio, F., and Kjellstrand, C.M. Association of Cancer with Primary Renal Disease. In: Rieselbach R.E. and Garnick, M.B., eds.: Cancer and the Kidney. Philadelphia: Lea and Febiger, 1982, p. 897.

3.  Bennington, J.L. and Beckwith, J.B.: Tumors of the kidney, renal pelvis, and ureter. In: Atlas of Tumor Pathology. Second Series, Fascicle 12. Washington, D.C., Armed Forces Institute of Pathology, 1975.

4.  Elliott, A.Y., et al.: Isolation of RNA virus from a papil- lary tumor of the human renal pelvis. Science 179:393, 1973.

5.  Olson, C., et al.: Oncogenicity of bovine papilloma virus. Arch. Environ. Health. 19:827, 1969.

6.  Petkovic, S.D.: A plea for conservative operation for ureteral tumors. J. Urol. 107:220, 1972.

7.  Bloom, N.A., Vidone, R.A., and Lytton, B.: Primary carcinoma of the ureter: A report of 102 new cases, J. Urol. 103:590, 1970.

8.  Grabstald, H., Whitmore, W.F., Jr., and Melamed, M.R.: Renal pelvic tumors. J.A.M.A. 218:845, 1971.

9.  Skinner, D.G., et al.: The clinical significance of carcinoma-in-situ of the urinary bladder and its association with overt carcinoma. J. Urol. 112:68, 1974.

10. Batata, M., and Grabstald, H.: Upper urinary tract urothelial tumors. Urol. Clin. North. Am. 3:79, 1976.

11. Jewett, H.J., and Strong, G.H.: Infiltrating carcinoma of the bladder: Relation of depth of penetration of the bladder wall to incidence of local extension and metastases. J. Urol. 55:366, 1946.

12. Almgard, L.E., Freedman, D., and Ljungqvist, A.: Carcinoma of the ureter with special reference to malignancy grading and prognosis. Scand. J. Urol. Nephrol. 7:165, 1973.

13. Bergman, H., Friedenberg, R.M., and Sayegh, V.: New roentgenologic signs of carcinoma of the ureter. Am, J. Roentgen. 86:707, 1961.

14. Casey, W.C., and Goodwin, W.E.: Percutaneous antegrade pyelography and hydronephrosis. J. Urol. 74:164, 1955.

15. Lang, E.K. and Norse, M.:  The roentgenographic diagnosis
    of obstuctive lesions of the ureter. J. Urol. 101:812,
    1969.

16. Cullen, T.H. Popham, R.R., and Voss, H.J.: Urine cytology
    and primary carcinoma of the renal pelvis and ureter.
    Aust. N.Z. J. Surg. 41:230, 1972.

17. Grace, D.A., et al.: Carcinoma of the renal pelvis: A 15
    year review. J. Urol. 98:566, 1967.

18. Zincke, H., et al.: Significance of urinary cytology in
    the early detection of transitional cell cancer of the
    upper urinary tract. J. Urol. 116:781, 1976.

19. Gill, W.B., Lu, C.T., and Thomasen, S.:  Retrograde
    brushing: A new technique for obtaining histologic and
    cytologic material from ureteral renal pelvic, and renal
    calyceal lesions. J. Urol. 109:573, 1973.

20. Blute R.D., Jr., Gittes R.S., and Gittes, R.F.:  Renal
    brush biopsy.  Survey of indications, techniques, and
    results. J. Urol. 126:146, 1981.

21. Strong, D.W., and Pearse, H.D.:  Recurrent urothelial
    tumors following surgery for transitional cell carcinoma
    of the upper urinary tract.  Cancer 38:2178, 1976.

22. McIntyre, D., Pyrah, L.N., and Raper, F.P.:  Primary
    ureteric neoplasms, with a report of forty cases. Br. J.
    Urol. 37:160, 1965.

23. Blute, R.D., Jr. and Richie, J.P.:  Tumors of the renal
    pelvis and ureter. J. Urol. In press, 1982.

24. Murphy, D.M., Zincke, H., and Furlow, W.L.:  Primary grade
    I transitional cell carcinoma of the renal pelvis and
    ureter. J. Urol. 123:629, 1980.

25. Batata, M.A., et al.:  Primary carcinoma of the ureter, a
    prognostic study. Cancer 35:1626, 1975.

26. Brady, L.W., et al.:  Radiation therapy, a valuable
    adjunct in the management of carcinoma of the ureter.
    J.A.M.A. 206:2871, 1968.

SECTION III


BLADDER CANCER


Carcinoma of the bladder allows the oncologist the opportunity to study in vivo long-term and latent effects of
various carcinogens excreted into and acting upon the transitional epithelium. The thoughtful analysis of natural history
highlights the salient features and elucidates some of the
problems inherent in decisions for appropriate therapy.
Advocates of surgery, radiation therapy, or combined modalities for treatment of invasive bladder cancer have fortified
their positions. The use of intravesical chemotherapy has
brought new promise for the patient at high risk of rapid
superficial recurrences and may be useful as well for the
patient with carcinoma in situ. Considerations in the selection of various chemotherapeutic agents for patients with
advanced bladder cancer have been updated. The multimodal
approach to childhood sarcomas, detailed in this section, has
improved survival rates considerably while minimizing
morbidity.

CHAPTER 11A

WILMS' TUMOR:  NATURAL HISTORY

J. Robert Cassady

I.  GENERAL

A.  Commonest primary renal tumor of childhood

B.  1-2 cases/$10^6$ population (around 400-500 cases/ yr. in U.S.)

C.  5-8% bilateral

II.  OTHER ASSOCIATED PROBLEMS

A.  Association with hemihypertrophy, aniridia (chromosome $11_q$), renal anomalies, other congenital anomalies (esp. bilateral cases), Von Recklinghausen's disease

B.  Frequency:  R side = L side

C.  Mean and median age: 3-1/2 yr.

D.  Mesoblastic nephroma - non-Wilms' tumor - usually present in less than 6 mo. old child - benign tumor requiring only surgical therapy

III.  SYMPTOMS

    A.  Abdominal mass (noted by parent)

    B.  Abdominal pain

    C.  Rarely, hematuria/hypertension

IV.  DIAGNOSTIC EVALUATION

    A.  History and physical

    B.  Chest PA and lateral, IVP

    C.  Ultrasound especially to note patency of IVC - if
        questionable, do I.V. cavagram

    D.  ? CT scan of lungs

    E.  CBC, urinalysis, liver function studies

    F.  Angiogram in selected cases

    G.  Bone scan in clear cell sarcoma patients

    H.  CT scan of brain in rhabdomyosarcomatous variety

V.  HISTOLOGY

    A.  Mesoblastic nephroma (see above - benign tumor)
        1.  "Common type" - 85%+ of cases
        2.  Anaplastic - 7-10% (adverse prognosis)
        3.  Sarcomatous varieties - 7-10% (adverse
           prognosis)

    B.  pre-malignant or in situ types; i.e. Wilms'
        tumorlet - seen especially with bilateral lesions

    C.  Wilms' tumor

VI. STAGING

    A. Prognostic features include primary tumor size, capsular involvement, nodal involvement, complete surgical removal, age, collecting system involvement, and histology

    B. Two major systems: Children's Hospital Medical Center and National Wilms' Tumor Study

VII. TREATMENT

    A. Transperitoneal nephrectomy for unilateral cases

    B. Postoperative radiation therapy for more locally advanced cases

    C. Routine postoperative chemotherapy – active agents: vincristine, actinomycin D, adriamycin, cytoxan

    D. Aggressive multimodality treatment for patients who present with or develop metastases and for those with bilateral disease

VII. RESULTS

    A. Overall 80–85% cure rate

    B. 50–70% of patients with metastases at presentation are cured

    C. 50% of deaths occur with 15% of patients with anaplastic

    D. 2/3 of patients with bilateral disease cured

IX. CURRENT STUDIES

    A. Is radiation therapy necessary in patients with NWTS stage II?

    B. What is optimal radiation dose for microscopic and gross disease?

C.  What is optimal combination and schedule of drugs?

D.  Contemplated study:  Is any postoperative therapy
    necessary for young patients with stage I disease?

SELECTED REFERENCES

1.  Beckwith, J.B. and Palmer, N.F.:  Histopathology and
    prognosis of Wilms' tumor:  Results from the First
    National Wilms' Tumor Study.  Cancer 41:1937, 1978.

2.  Cassady, J.R., et al:  Considerations in the treatment of
    Wilms' tumor.  Cancer 32:598, 1973.

3.  Leape, L.L., Breslow, N.E. and Bishop, H.C.:  The surgical
    treatment of Wilms' tumor:  Results of the National Wilms'
    Tumor Study.  Ann. Surg. 187:  351, 1978.

4.  Breslow, N.E., et al.:  Wilms' tumor:  Prognostic factors
    for patients without metastases at diagnosis.  Cancer
    41:1577, 1978.

5.  Bove, K.F. and McAdams, A.J.:  The nephroblastomatosis
    complex and its relationship to Wilms' tumor:  a clinico-
    pathologic treatise.  In:  Rosenberg, H.S. and Bolande,
    R.P., eds.:  Perspectives in Pediatric Pathology, vol. 3.
    Chicago: Year Book Med.  Publishers, 1976, pp. 185.

6.  Cassady, J.R. and Jaffe, N.:  Wilms' tumor:  controversies
    on current forms of management.  In:  Carter, S.K.,
    Glastein, E., Livingston, R.B., eds.:  Principles of Cancer
    Treatment.  New York: McGraw-Hill, 1982, pp.847.

CHAPTER 11B

WILMS' TUMOR: SURGICAL ASPECTS

Judah Folkman

I.  CLINICAL PRESENTATION

Wilms' tumor is the second most common intra-abdominal
malignant solid tumor in children (after neuroblastoma).
The tumor presents as an abdominal mass usually in a child
under five years of age.  The mass has most often been
noted by a parent, and the patient may complain of intermittent abdominal pain.  Asymptomatic hematuria or fever
is present in about one-third of the patients.  Most
Wilms' tumors are sufficiently large at the time of presentation that it is not possible to separate them from
the costal margin with one's hand.  After the first abdominal examination, we try to limit subsequent abdominal
examinations to only those absolutely necessary in an
attempt to avoid compression of the tumor and possible
release of tumor thrombi.

II. PREOPERATIVE EVALUATION

A.  An abdominal ultrasound to show that the mass is
solid and to see if the vena cava contains tumor
thrombus.

B.  An intravenous pyelogram that shows calyceal distortion rather than displacement is virtually diagnostic of Wilms' tumor.

81

C.  An angiogram is not usually obtained, unless the diagnosis is still in doubt, e.g. a liver tumor that overlies the right kidney.

D.  A chest x-ray, computed tomographic scan of the whole lung and a liver scan to determine the extent of metastases.  Bone marrow aspiration and biopsy have a low yield and are not usually indicated preoperatively. The patient is cross-matched for sufficient blood for at least one blood volume.

E.  A venacavagram is done if the ultrasound is in doubt.  An echocardiogram is obtained if tumor thrombus extends above the diaphragm.


III.   POSITIONING IN THE OPERATING ROOM

A.  A Foley catheter is inserted.  Cystoscopy may be advisable if there has been gross hematuria in order to determine if tumor protrudes from a ureter.

B.  Two intravenous lines are placed in the upper extremities, or one in the neck and one in the arm.  Leg veins are avoided because the vena cava may become obstructed during manipulation of the tumor.

C.  A small kidney roll is placed beneath the flank, and the patient is turned upward about 30 degrees in the supine position.  The arm on the side of the lesion is placed over the head so that an incision can be carried into the chest if necessary.

D.  A nasogastric tube is passed and placed on suction.

E.  A cautery plate is placed.

F.  For all children, it is wise to have a heating blanket in place.


IV.   INTRA-OPERATIVE PROCEDURE (EXCISION OF WILMS' TUMOR)

A.  The patient is prepped and draped from nipples to pubis to expose the chest on the side of the lesion.

B.  The surgeon should have at least two assistants.

C.  A transabdominal incision is made in the upper
abdomen.  It should cross both rectus muscles and extend
almost to the mid-axillary line on the side of the
lesion.  It is only very rarely that one has to extend
the incision into the chest through the costal margin at
about the eighth interspace.  Nearly all tumors I have
encountered can be removed through this intra-abdominal
incision.

D.  The transverse colon is usually draped over the
tumor, and its mesentery must be dissected free.  The
tumor does not usually invade the mesentery so that
there is a free plane.  At the end of the procedure, it
is important to check the mesentery and repair all holes
in it, since these have been the site of post-operative
small bowel obstruction.

E.  For right-sided lesions, a Kocher maneuver to mobil-
ize the duodenum is important at this point.  For a
large tumor, it is rarely possible to isolate the renal
vessels until late in the procedure.

F.  The small intestine is packed off away from the
tumor.

G.  As one dissects, three rules are kept in mind.

   1.  Dissection follows the curve of the tumor, but
       stays in the plane just superficial to the
       serpentiginous veins that cover the surface of
       the tumor.

   2.  The tumor is gently lifted rather than leaned
       upon.

   3.  One tries to avoid spill or rupture.

H. It is usually easiest to begin dissection laterally,
working as far under the tumor as possible until one can
begin to lift the tumor.  This permits the dissection to
continue inferiorly.  Placing a hand beneath the tumor
to thin out the structures at the lower pole of the
tumor is helpful.  This maneuver also protects the iliac
vein.

I.  Dissection then continues from the lower pole
medially.  At this time the ureter may be dissected
free.

J.  If the upper pole of the tumor has not invaded the
liver (i.e., a free plane exists between the tumor and
the liver), the upper pole is dissected.  If tumor
invades the liver, this portion of the operation is
deferred until after the renal vessels have been ligated
and divided so that the kidney can be lifted up and a
partial hepatectomy can be performed as a wedge resection of the liver.

K.  After both poles are freed, it is safe to begin to
isolate the renal vessels.  The tumor should be lifted
gently and moved medially.  Tenting of the vena cava is
a danger here.  It is important to visualize the connec-
tion of the renal vein with the cava so that the
opposite renal vein is not pulled over and clamped inad-
vertantly.  The same precaution is taken with the renal
artery.  However, to get to these vessels, one usually
has to ligate several large feeder veins which extend
from the tumor to the lumbar vessels and occassionally
"stand guard" around the main renal vessels.  One
usually tries to ligate and divide the renal artery
first.  I prefer to avoid placing any clamps on the
renal artery in order to prevent avulsion from the
aorta.  Instead, a tie is placed proximally on the renal
artery and one distally, and then a suture ligature is
placed between these, closer to the proximal tie,
leaving room to transect the renal artery.

L.  The renal vein is then dissected free and tran-
sected in the same way.  However, if there is any
indication of clot in the renal vein (i.e., left-sided
variocele seen preoperatively, thrombi noted on ultrasound or cavagram, proteinuria, or gross appearance of
thrombus in the vein) then it is wise to place a
Satinsky or Potts curved vascular clamp across the vein
before transecting it.

M.  Removal of tumor thrombus from the vein.  Two fine
cardiovascular sutures (4-0 or 5-0) are placed at the
tip of the vein to hold it on tension.  The clamp is
removed while the anesthetist provides positive inspiratory pressure.  This maneuver will often expel

thrombus. If not, the thrombus can be pulled from the cava with a ring forceps or a small gallstone common duct clamp or suctioned. It is rare for the tumor thrombus to break up. It is usually connected over a long stretch by tumor blood vessels. There may be tumor in the opposite renal vein (pre-operative intravenous pyelogram with reduced or absent function bilaterally). If tumor thrombus remains in the cava and extends above the diaphragm, cardiac bypass will be required to prevent fatal pulmonary embolism. Under cardiopulmonary bypass the right artrium is opened and tumor is removed from above and below the diaphragm. Two such patients have been successfully treated at the Children's Hospital in Boston during the past two years.

N. The ureter is dissected as close to the bladder as possible and then ligated and divided with catgut sutures. The end is examined to make sure that it does not contain tumor.

O. Gerota's fascia is opened over the opposite kidney, which is bimanually palpated to determine if any tumors are present. Bilateral disease occurs in five percent of Wilms' tumor cases, is often multi-focal and associated with other congenital anomalies, appears in younger patients of older mothers, has a lower incidence of pulmonary metastasis, and has a more favorable cure rate of about 85 percent. Based on these facts, a single lower pole lesion in the opposite kidney could be resected from the kidney. However, multiple small lesions are left alone as they will respond well to subsequent chemotherapy.

P. The para-aortic nodes are examined and the highest node may be excised if only for staging purposes. However, a node dissection is usually not done, as there is no evidence that it increases survival rate.

Q. If tumor spill occurs, it should, if possible, be walled off from the general peritoneal cavity. Tumor spill does not adversely affect prognosis if it is appropriately treated with irradiation of the whole abdomen.

R. A tear in the renal vein or vena cava is the most serious problem than can arise during dissection of a large renal tumor, especially since the renal vein may be splayed or flattened by tumor beneath it. This can be handled in one of three ways:

1. Pressure over the tear with a large square of teflon felt. After about 5 to 6 minutes when pressure is released, the felt will hold in place over the tear allowing blood flow through the vein. The felt may be left in place and trimmed, or carefully lifted from one corner while sutures are placed.

2. Application of blunt Allis clamps to the tear after which a continuous vascular suture is placed as each clamp is removed one at a time.

3. In life-threatening hemorrhage, when there is a large tear in the cava, the abdomen fills with blood, and cardiac arrest is imminent, the best maneuver is to quickly hyperextend the table (or in an emergency, reach beneath the patient and lift up under the back) so that the feet and the head almost touch the floor. This causes blood to stand in the veins of the extremities and in the veins of the chest, and at the same time forces the spine to compress the cava so that one can in fact see the hole in the cava. The cava can then be quickly sutured or cross clamped, and the patient returned to the normal position.

S. Postoperative complications. Intestinal obstruction may occur early from an adhesion or later from radiation ileitis. When a large tumor on the right has been removed and the tumor bed irradiated, the patient may develop more toxic symptoms from chemotherapy than from a left-sided tumor. This is thought to be due to mild radiation hepatitis on the right side. Small children under two years of age who require total abdominal radiation will almost invariably need intravenous hyperalimentation for part of their postoperative course. Otherwise, Wilms' tumor patients do well, and once the nasogastric tube is removed, they are able to ambulate and leave the hospital within 1 to 2 weeks.

T.  Late metastasis.  Isolated lung metastasis may
appear several years after chemotherapy and radiotherapy
have been completed.  These are best treated by thoraco-
tomy and wedge resection usually followed by whole lung
radiation.

U.  If pulmonary metastases are present at the time of
initial excision of the abdominal tumor, one of these
may be removed by wedge biopsy of the lung so that
appropriate chemotherapy and radiotherapy can be planned
for the postoperative period.

SUGGESTED REFERENCES

1.  Malcolm, A.W., et al.:  Bilateral Wilms' tumor.  Int. J.
    Rad. Oncol. Biol. Phy. 6:167, 1980.

2.  Leape, L.L., Breslow, N.E. and Bishop, H.C.:  The surgical
    treatment of Wilms' tumor - Results of the National Wilms'
    Tumor Study.  Ann. Surg. 187:351, 1978.

3.  Schullinger, J.N., et al.:  Wilms' tumor:  The role of
    right heart angiography in the management of selected
    cases.  Ann. Surg.  185:451, 1977.

4.  Jereb, B., et al.:  Lymph node invasion and prognosis in
    nephroblastoma.  Cancer 45:1632, 1980.

5.  Keep, C.E.:  Current management of nephroblastoma and
    neuroblastoma.  Am. J. Surg. 107:497, 1964.

6.  Green, D.M. and Jaffe, N.:  Wilms' tumor - Model of a
    curable pediatric solid tumor.  Cancer Treat. Rev. 5:
    143, 1978.

CHAPTER 11C

WILMS' TUMOR: CHEMOTHERAPY

Stephen E. Sallan

A.  GENERAL CONSIDERATIONS

1.  The tumor is sensitive to at least four drugs

        Vincristine
        Actinomycin D
        Adriamycin
        Cyclophosphamide

2.  Combinations of two (or more) drugs are more effective than single agents.

3.  Multiple courses of the combinations are superior to a single course
    a.  The "optimal" duration of treatment is under continuous investigation.

4.  The choice of drugs and duration of treatment depend on two features.
    a.  Extent of disease (Stage)
    b.  Histopathology

B.  APPROACHES TO TREATMENT

1.  Babies (under 2 years old) with small, completely resectable tumors of favorable histopathology (FH)

89

    a.  Nephrectomy
    b.  No radiation therapy
    c.  Maximum of 6 months chemotherapy with vincristine
        and actinomycin D
    d.  Comment - it is possible that such patients, if
        meticulously staged to exclude any adverse prog-
        nostic feature, may not require chemotherapy.

2.  Older children (over 2 years old) with small tumor,
    of FH

    a.  Nephrectomy
    b.  Vincristine and actinomycin D for 6 months
    c.  Comment - controversy exist whether size, per se,
        should influence therapy in this group; larger
        tumors may increase the risk of tumor bed recur-
        rences in unirradiated patients.

3.  Patients of any age with larger tumors of FH
    (without distant metastases)

    a.  Nephrectomy
    b.  Tumor bed radiotherapy
    c.  Vincristine and actinomycin D (+ adriamycin)
    d.  Comments - if tumor has "spilled" beyond capsule,
        radiotherapy should include whole abdomen; the
        value of the addition of adriamycin to these
        patients remains controversial.

4.  Patients with pulmonary metastases and either FH or
    unfavorable histopathology (UH)

    a.  Nephrectomy
    b.  Local and whole lung radiotherapy
    c.  Vincristine and actinomycin D and a third drug
        (either cyclophosphamide or adriamycin)
    d.  Comment - the choice of chemotherapy is compli-
        cated by the known additive cardiotoxicity of
        adriamycin and radiation.

5.  Patients with non-metastatic tumors of UH

    a.  Nephrectomy
    b.  Radiotherapy
    c.  Vincristine and actinomycin D and a third drug
        (either cyclophosphamide or adriamycin)

    d.  Comment — these are unusual patients and guide-
        lines are less certain

  6.  Patients with extra-pulmonary metastases or bilateral
     disease

    a.  Individualize using principles from either groups
        of patients.


C.  STUDIES

  1. National Wilms' Tumor Study (NWTS) Study I,
     1969–1974, showed that:
     1. local radiotherapy was unnecessary in Group I
        patients under 2 years old if chemotherapy was
        given;
     2. that older patients had local recurrences without
        radiotherapy;
     3. combination chemotherapy was superior to single
        agent; an 4) pre-operative chemotherapy was
        unnecessary.

  2.  NWTS II Study II, 1974–1978, showed that:
     1. in patients with resectable tumors limited to the
        kidney, radiotherapy was unnecessary if the combi-
        nation of vincristine and actinomycin D was used
        for at least 6 months;
     2. in the above patients, 6 months of chemotherapy
        were as effective as 15 months;
     3. the addition of adriamycin to vincristine and acti-
        nomycin D resulted in better relapse-free survival
        than the latter two drug combination in patients
        with more advanced disease;
     4. unfavorable histopathology and lymph node involve-
        ment were of adverse prognostic importance.

  3.  Green and Jaffe.  This retrospective study showed
     that:
     1. in babies under 2 years old with small tumors,
        nephrectomy alone is as effective as nephrectomy
        and radiotherapy plus chemotherapy;
     2. the addition of postoperative radiotherapy and
        adjuvant single agent chemotherapy did not

improve relapse-free survival in patients with
resectable limited tumors who had no metastatic
disease; and:
3. for that group, combination chemotherapy (vincristine and actinomycin D) improved disease-free
survival.

SUGGESTED REFERENCES


1. D'Angio, G.J., et al.: The treatment of Wilms' tumor:
   Results of the National Wilms' Tumor Study. Cancer
   38:633, 1976.

2. D'Angio, G.J., et al.: The treatment of Wilms' tumor:
   Results of Second National Wilms' Tumor Study. Cancer
   47:2302, 1981.

3. Green, D.M. and Jaffe, N.: The role of chemotherapy in
   the treatment of Wilms' tumor. Cancer 44:52, 1979.

4. Morris-Jones, P.H. et al.: Management of nephroblastoma
   in childhood. Arch. Dis. Child. 53:112, 1978.

CHAPTER 12

BLADDER CANCER - NATURAL HISTORY

Leonard N. Zinman

Cancer of the bladder accounts for 2% of all malignant
disease. Most tumors of the bladder are transitional cell
carcinomas (92%) with a 6% to 7% incidence of squamous cell
carcinoma and a 1% to 2% incidence of adenocarcinoma.
Non-epithelial tumors include sarcoma, pheochromocytoma,
malignant lymphoma, mixed mesodermal tumor, and primary carcinoid. Transitional cell carcinoma usually is localized at
the time of initial diagnosis with a 9% incidence of regional
metastases and a 6% incidence of distant metastases. The
incidence of the disease is 20 per 100,000 in persons over age
40, increases with age to an incidence of 150 per 100,000 at
age 70, and has a male to female predominance of 2 to 1.

Optimal management of cancer of the bladder depends on an
accurate understanding of the stage in which it presents, the
natural history of that stage, and the variables that help
predict the course of the individual tumor. Much of this
critical information is either fragmentary or not yet available. Most patients with bladder cancer have a protracted
clinical course with a long history of carcinoma-in-situ or
multiple recurrences of superficial tumors preceding the
invasive disease. A smaller group of patients (20% to 25%)
appear at onset with an invasive lesion that progresses
rapidly and is not altered by any form of therapy. This
malignancy is probably a heterogeneous group of tumors that
have a varied clinical course influenced by such poorly under-
stood factors as host-tumor immune response, pre-existing or
associated carcinoma-in-situ disease, morphology, rapidity of
recurrence of prior tumors,and iatrogenic factors, such as
transurethral resection. irrigating fluids, mucosal trauma,

chemotherapy, and radiotherapy.


PREDICTIVE STUDIES

The key factor in determining virulence is the stage or
extent of depth into the bladder wall that a tumor reaches.
Increasing weight has been given to grade and the presence of
associated carcinoma-in-situ in adjacent or distant mucosa,
since considerable error has been made in attempting to determine accurately the level of disease in the muscle. The five-
year survival of B1 and B2 disease is similar, ranging from
40% to 50% in most series. Once muscle invasion has been
identified, therapy should be based on muscle involvement
rather than on attempts made to separate various levels. The
cumulative error in understaging is 40% to 75% with a 30%
error in overstaging on T2/T3 lesions. Chisholm et al. have
also suggested a single invasive category, T2 to T3, as being
more practical since the biologic behavior of clinical T2 and
T3 is similar in their experience.

Bergkvist and associates demonstrated a good correlation
between the grade of the tumor and survival in patients
observed for more than eight years. Mortality increased from
0% for grade I to 50% for grade II and 90% for grade III
lesions during the period of observation. For many years, it
has been demonstrated that for the most part grade and stage
go hand in hand. Low-grade tumors are encountered in superficial stages, and high-grade tumors are associated with deep
invasion with only an 8% deviation from this general observation. The grading has been a modified version of the Broders'
classification (grades I to III) since the behavior of grade
III and grade IV have been found to be almost identical.

The second area of interest relevant to predicting potential for bladder tumor progression is that associated with
superficial tumors. It is now recognized that multiplicity in
time and space, grade, and associated carcinoma-in-situ are
all strong predictors of the development of invasive disease.

It has been difficult, however, to distinguish histologically benign papillomas from malignant epithelial tumors.
Results of a survey of 125 patients with papillomas observed
for 11 months to 20 years indicated a 16.2% incidence of
development of true subsequent bladder cancer over a five-year
period, but the five-year survival for papilloma is

essentially the same as the five-year expectancy of general
age- matched population.

Chromosomal markers and blood group antigens on the tumor
cell surface are other predictors to determine tumor virulence
and to predict biologic potential of tumors of the bladder. A
tumor with an absent marker chromosome and a tumor with intact
cell surface blood group antigens have a more benign nature
and a better prognosis. These two techniques appear to have
close correlation but require considerable skill to perform
with reproducible results.

The incidence of the various stages and grades of tumor is
difficult to determine since the reports from various centers
reflect a selection of patients based on certain referral
patterns. In a review of 270 unselected new patients from the
United Kingdom presenting with bladder tumors, 39% were T1,
26% were T2, 28% were T3, and 6% were T4. The size of the
tumor was less than 3 cm in 37% of the patients, 3 to 5 cm in
30%, and more than 5 cm in 33% of patients. Of the entire
group, 63% presented with multiple lesions. The incidence of
lymph node involvement varies from different surgical units
depending on whether or not there has been previous radiation.
In the non-radiated patient, there is a 5% to 10% incidence of
lymph node involvement in P1 and P in situ lesions, 30% in P2
and 40% in the P3 category. In the National Bladder Cancer
Collaborative study, these figures were at variance with a 48%
incidence of mucosal disease (Ta), 31% incidence of lamina
propria (T1), and a 21% incidence of T2 and T3 disease.


CARCINOMA-IN-SITU

The definition of carcinoma in situ has been changed
recently to include papillary epithelial lesions. Common
usage, however, implies a flat intraepithelial lesion, with a
severe degree of anaplasia (grade III) and with a loss of cell
cohesiveness that accounts for a high incidence of abnormal
cytology. The two forms of this disease are focal and diffuse. Diffuse is the commoner form and is often associated
with an overt tumor. When it occurs without macroscopic bladder cancer, the incidence of microinvasive disease at the time
of cystectomy is 20%. When the diffuse form is seen in
patients with a history of bladder cancer, the likelihood of
an invasive tumor developing is 42%. The presence of
carcinoma-in-situ in close proximity to a superficial bladder

tumor is predictive of an 83% chance that an invasive tumor
will ultimately develop. Diffuse involvement of the bladder
is usual, with the lower half of the bladder the commoner
location of the lesion. The vesical neck and proximal urethra
are involved in 60% of the cases; a high incidence of
progression into the periurethral prostatic ducts is evident
in this latter group. The distal ureters are involved in over
50% of bladders possessing diffuse carcinoma-in-situ.

Irritative bladder symptoms, histologic evidence of
disease into the ureters, vesical neck, and urethra, and
persistent biopsy or cytologic evidence of disease after 6 to
12 months of chemotherapy are predictive factors in identifying future invasive disease. Patients with incidentally
discovered in situ cancer seem to have a more focal variety of
the disease, which uncommonly progresses to invasion.

Industrial bladder cancer has a similar natural history.
Three distinct periods of development of the cancer were
recognized. Firstly, a latent period of a few months to eight
years exists after exposure to xenylamine when histology and
cytology are normal. Then, a period of a few months to 11
years in which a positive cytology developed, followed by a
period of 6 months to 2 years during which invasive cancer
developed in 7 of 13 patients. Two patients had reversal of
their cytology to normal.


SUPERFICIAL BLADDER CANCER: Ta, T1

Of the newly diagnosed cases followed by the National
Bladder Cancer Collaborative Group A, 198 of 259 fell into the
Ta, T1 category. The distribution of grade was 35% grade I,
35% grade II, and 30% grade III. Of the 120 patients with
mucosal disease (Ta), only 4 (3.3%) went on to have muscle
invasion, whereas 25% of the patients (78) with a T1 tumor
developed muscle invasion within a two-year period. If the T1
tumor was a grade III, there was a 40% chance of muscle
invasion over the same period of observation.

The presence of severe dysplasia or carcinoma-in-situ
increased the likelihood of muscle invasion but not as much as
originally believed. The other two factors associated with
progression were the size of the tumor and an increase in
grade with each recurrence.

In general, low-grade, small, solitary tumors that did not
have distant dysplasia were at minimal risk for recurrence.
For the entire group studied, the median time for first recurrence was 31 months compared to 13 months from the successful
treatment of a first recurrence to a diagnosis of a second
recurrence and 12 months from second to third.


INVASIVE TUMORS: T2, T3

Invasive bladder cancer is probably a mixed heterogeneous
group of tumors with some characteristics that may actually
identify their potential virulence.  These characteristics
include response to radiotherapy, involvement of perivesical
fat, lymphatics, vascular invasion, prostatic or nodal
extension, degree of differentiation, and whether a tumor is
solid or papillary.  A poor prognosis now is well known to
correlate with histologic proof of lymphatic invasion.  Of 10
patients with lymphatic involvement in stage T1 disease, 7
died of metastatic disease within six years, testifying to the
relevance of this finding.  Survival rates for invasive
bladder cancer have varied over the past two decades with each
modality of therapy.  Surgical extirpation results in a five-
year survival of 9% to 31%; radiation, 19% to 33%; and
combined radiation and cystectomy, 35% to 52%.  Local recurrence with cystectomy occurs in 30% to 45% of patients, and
local failure with radiation alone is 39% to 45%.  Only 35% to
50% of the patients with deeply infiltrating tumors will
survive a five-year period since distant metastases will
develop in 30% to 50% in a 12- to 18-month period after
initial diagnosis.  Within a 10- to 12-week period after
diagnosis, 5% to 10% of these patients will go from stage
T2/T3 to T4 disease.

Radiotherapy will downstage all stages of invasive disease
from 32% to 40% irrespective of the depth of invasion.  There
is complete eradication of the tumor in 25% to 30% of
patients, and in general, this group of patients has a 20%
improvement in five-year survival over patients who do not
respond to radiation.  Patients classified as C or D1 and
those with a palpable mass do not have a change in survival
pattern even with downstaging response to radiation.  Papillary tumors have a much better response to radiation than
solid tumors with a 30% versus a 42% incidence of tumor in the
surgical specimen.  Responses to radical radiotherapy reveal a
40% complete response over a 3- to 6-month period (32 of 81),

partial response in 23% (19 of 81), and none in 37% (30 of
81). The size of the invasive tumor has some impact on
survival with a 40% three-year survival in tumors less than
5 cm compared to a 20% survival in those with larger tumors if
treated by radical radiotherapy. No difference is noted in
groups undergoing both radiotherapy and cystectomy. The
five-year survival for radiotherapy alone is 19% to 33% with
one exception, the report from Bloom et al. at the London
Hospital revealing a five-year survival of 38%.

     Combined cystectomy and preoperative radiotherapy survival
figures look better than any other modality, but most studies
have not been well controlled. These range from 34% to 53%
with an average five-year survival rate of 40% for T3
disease. It may be that withdrawal of patients from the
combined treatment arms due to inoperability at the time of
surgery will lead to some bias in favor of preoperative
radiation. The removal of patients undergoing salvage
cystectomy from the radical radiotherapy arm is also
unfavorable to the radiotherapy group, since results of late
cystectomy were good and also bias the results in favor of the
combined treatment. Lymph node disease occurs in 40% to 50%
of patients with deeply invasive bladder cancer. If they have
stage reduction after radiation therapy, metastatic disease to
the lymph nodes decreases to 5% to 10% as opposed to 35% of
patients with radioresistant tumor. These factors suggest the
presence of different categories of bladder cancer based on
responses to radiation therapy. A considerable variation in
the natural history of invasive disease is evident in the
various subgroups, with a 14% to 74% three-year survival
depending upon the response to radiation therapy. The
incidence of pelvic recurrence is lower with the combined
method amounting to 18% to 20% vs 37% after cystectomy alone.


METASTATIC DISEASE

     Extension of invasive bladder cancer beyond the bladder
into pelvic lymph nodes (D1) is usually the harbinger of
distant metastases. This stage should also include invasion
of the pelvic wall, rectus muscles below the umbilicus, and
adjacent organs, such as prostate, cervix, or vagina.
Although there has been reported as much as a 17% incidence of
survival in patients with one or two positive nodes, this has
not consistently been confirmed. Tumor that invades directly
into the prostatic stroma has been associated with rare

survival and should clearly be distinguished from superficial
transitional cell tumor found in the periurethral prostatic
ducts.

SUGGESTED REFERENCES

1.  Althausen, A.F., Prout G.R., Jr. and Daly, J.J.:
    Non-invasive papillary carcinoma of the bladder
    associated with carcinoma in situ. J. Urol. 116:575,
    1976.

2.  Anderson, C.K.: Current topics in the pathology of
    bladder cancer. Proc. Roy. Soc. Med. 66:283, 1973.

3.  Bergkvist, A., Ljungqvist, A. and Moberger, G.:
    Classification of bladder tumours based on the cellular
    pattern. Preliminary report of a clinical-pathological
    study of 300 cases with a minimum follow-up of eight
    years. Acta Chir. Scand. 130:371, 1965.

4.  Bloom, H.J.G., et al.: Treatment of T3 bladder cancer:
    Controlled trial of pre-operative radiotherapy and
    radical cystectomy versus radical radiotherapy. Br. J.
    Urol. 54:136, 1982.

5.  Chisholm, G.D., et al.: TNM (1978) in bladder cancer:
    use and abuse. Br. J. Urol. 52:500, 1980.

6.  England, H.R., Paris A.M. and Blandy, J.P.: The
    correlation of T1 bladder tumour history with prognosis
    and follow-up requirements. Br. J. Urol. 53:593, 1981.

7.  Farrow, G.M., et al.: Clinical observations on
    sixty-nine cases of in situ carcinoma of the urinary
    bladder. Canc. Res. 37:2794, 1977.

8.  Gilbert, H.A., et al.: The natural history of papillary
    transitional cell carcinoma of the bladder and its
    treatment in an unselected population on the basis of
    histological grading. J. Urol. 119:488, 1978.

9.  LaPlante, M. and Brice, M.: The upper limits of hopeful
    application of radical cystectomy for vesical
    carcinoma: does nodal metastasis always indicate
    incurability? J. Urol. 109:261, 1973.

10. Lerman, R.I., Hutter, R.V.P. and Whitmore, W.F., Jr.:
    Papilloma of the urinary bladder. Cancer 25:333, 1970.

11. Melamed, M.R., Voutsa, N.G. and Grabstald, H.: Natural
    history and clinical behavior of in situ carcinoma of
    the human urinary bladder. Cancer 17:1533, 1964.

12. Miller, A., Mitchell, J.P. and Brown, N.J.: The Bristol
    Bladder Tumour Registry. Br. J. Urol. 41:Suppl:1, 1969.

13. Mostofi, F.K.: Study of 2678 patients with initial
    carcinoma of the bladder: I. Survival rates. J. Urol.
    75:480, 1956.

14. Newman, A.J., Jr., Carlton, C.E., Jr. and Johnson, S.:
    Cell surface A, B, or O(H) blood group antigens as an
    indicator of malignant potential in stage A bladder
    carcinoma. J. Urol. 124:27, 1980.

15. Prout, G.R., Griffin, P.A. and Shipley, W.U.: Bladder
    carcinoma as a systemic disease. Cancer 43:2532, 1979.

16. Skinner, D.G.: Current state of classification and
    staging of bladder cancer. Cancer Res. 37:2838, 1977.

17. Skinner, D.G., et al.: The clinical significance of
    carcinoma in situ of the bladder and its association
    with overt carcinoma. J. Urol. 112:68, 1974.

18. Soloway, M.S., et al.: Serial multiple-site biopsies in
    patients with bladder cancer. J. Urol. 120:57, 1978.

19. Thelmo. W.L., et al.: Carcinoma in situ of the bladder
    with associated prostatic involvement. J. Urol.
    111:491, 1974.

CHAPTER 13

INTRAVESICAL CHEMOTHERAPY FOR SUPERFICIAL BLADDER CARCINOMA

Marc B. Garnick

I  NATURAL HISTORY AND STAGING

The natural history of transitional cell carcinoma of the bladder that is superficial and limited to the mucosa or lamina propria is extremely variable. While 5 year survivorship ranges between 65-85%, 50-70% of patients will develop recurrent lesions of a similar or different stage and grade, as seen in Table 13-1.

Table 13-1. Superficial Bladder Cancer

| N | Disease Free p TUR/Fulg. | Relapse |
|---|---|---|
| 274 | 263 (96%) | 139 (51%) |

In a detailed natural history study by the National Bladder Cancer Collaborative Group A (Table 13-2) 21% (15 of 73 patients) with stage A ($T_1$) lesions developed muscle invasion over a 3 year period of time.

Table 13-2  Bladder Cancer - Natural History

| Stage | N | Progression to Deeper Layers |
|---|---|---|
| 0 | 175 | 10 ( 6%) |
| A | 73 | 15 (21%) |

101

While the likelihood of muscle invasion was less with stage $T_a$, a poorly differentiated grade had a substantial incidence of muscle invasion.

When considering treatment strategies for the management of superficial bladder carcinoma, the variables listed in Table 2 must be considered in terms of trying to identify patients at high risk for developing a more poorly differentiated lesion, or lesions which will become invasive.

Table 13-3.   Important Prognostic Variables

- Histopathology (TCC, squamous, adenocarcinoma)
- Pathologic grade
- Cellular atypia/Ca-in-situ
- Anatomic location
- Multiplicity of lesions
- Cytogenetic abnormalities
- Surface ABH antigens

The fact that traditional endoscopic resection of these superficial lesions is still accompanied by a substantial number of recurrences underscores the need for additional therapy to:
1. Decrease the number of recurrences.
2. Increase the duration between recurrences.
3. Decrease the likelihood of subsequent muscle and lymphatic invasion and ultimately disseminated spread.
4. To eradicate the disease completely.

Intravesical administration of antineoplastic agents has been used in the management of superficial bladder carcinoma. The rationale underlying its use includes:
1. The elimination of multifocal microscopic foci of cancer.
2. The elimination of pre-neoplastic and carcinoma-in-situ changes, two elements which are believed to be important in the pathogenesis of new and invasive lesions.
3) The ability to achieve high regional drug concentrations of the bladder mucosa and lamina propria.
4) The minimizing of systemic toxicity by selecting agents

which have minimal absorption through the bladder mucosa.

## II. INTRAVESICAL (IVe) CHEMOTHERAPEUTIC AGENTS

### A. Thiotepa and Epodyl Trials

Table 13-4.  IVe Therapy-Definitive Thiotepa

| Series | N | % CR | % PR | % Overall |
|--------|----|------|------|-----------|
| Pavone—Macaluso | 25 | 32 | 32 | 64 |
| Veenema | 46 | 37 | 35 | 72 |
| Koontz | 95 | 47 | -- | 47 |

Table 13-5.  IVe Therapy Trials

| Group | Study | N | Result |
|-------|-------|---|--------|
| EORTC randomized | Thiotepa VM 26 Control | $215(T_1)$ | Thiotepa decreased recurrence rate (p = .04) No difference in time to first recurrence |
| UK | Epodyl | 51 | 33% CR   Not randomized 39% PR 16% irritative symptoms |

### B. Prophylactic Trials with Thiotepa

There are now a number of trials looking at the use of intravesical chemotherapy in a prophylactic fashion.  Patients entered in these trials have been endoscopically rendered disease free, and then placed on chemotherapeutic agents with hopes of decreasing the number of recurrences or the time to recurrences after thiotepa.  Most investigations have demonstrated both of these factors when chemotherapy has been used in a prophylactic fashion.  In one such study, the efficacy of 30 or 60 mg of thiotepa administered intravesically monthly was compared with controls.  The percentage of patients who were tumor free at 12 and 20 months was greater for the thiotepa treated patients than for controls (66%

versus 40% and 54% versus 28%, p = .02).  Other comparative
trials have borne out the same types of information.

C.   Adriamycin

Table 13-6.  IVe Therapy with Adriamycin - Various Trials

| Dose(mg) | Schedule | Dwell Time | N | Results |
|---|---|---|---|---|
| 10 | weekly x4 then monthly | | 20 | 30% recurrence |
| 20-30 | TIW x 2 w. | | 194 | 31-56% RR* 31% SE+ |
| 50 | " | | | 68-72% RR  27% SE |
| 60 | " | | | 59-74% RR  44% SE |
| 80 | monthly | 1 hr. | 8 | 87% cysto - 17% SE |
| 40 vs. control | monthly | | 30 | 13/15 (87%) control had recurrence 5/15 (33%) ADR had recurrence |

*RR - response rate
+SE - side effects (usually consisting of dysuria, frequency,
bladder spasms).

D.   Adriamycin Experience at the Sidney Farber Cancer
     Institute and Brigham and Women's Hospital
     (Experience in 27 patients treated
     prophylactically - See Figure 13-1).

Table 13-7.  Response and Duration

| $T_a$, $T_1$ | N (%) |
|---|---|
| Complete Response (no recurrence; negative cytology) | 15/27 (55) |
| Failure (recurrence) | 7/27 (26) |
| Persistent Class V cytology Ca-in-situ | 3/27 (11) |
| Progressive disease | 1 (4) |
| Class V cytology | 1 (4) |
| Duration | |
| Median (range, months) | 12 (6-24) |

E.   Mitomycin-C

Recent studies have reported a 44% complete, and 32%

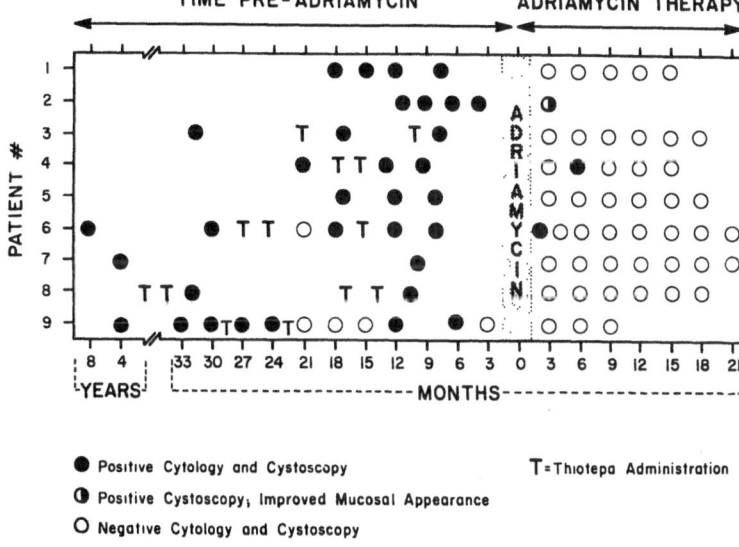

Figure 13-1.   Data in 9 Representative Patients


partial response rate in 50 patients receiving intravesical mitomycin-C in a dose of 20 mg.  A recently reported experience with mitomycin-C described the development of prostatic transitional cell carcinoma when the drug has been used for carcinoma-in-situ of the bladder.

F.    Miscellaneous Agents

A variety of other agents have been used for the management of superficial transitional cell carcinoma of the bladder. BCG immunotherapy using 120 mg of the Pasteur strain of BCG intravesically and 5 mg percutaneously has been evaluated versus control.  Overall, in this one large experience, 15/68 (22%) patients in the control group developed cystoscopic evidence of recurrent tumor, versus 6/84 (7%) patients in the BCG group.


III. CARCINOMA-IN-SITU

Two recent reports have emphasized the invasive potential of carcinoma-in-situ, especially in that group of patients who

are treated conservatively. Both investigators have stressed
the need for prompt cystectomy in the subset of patients who
are early failures on intravesical chemotherapy for carcinoma-
in-situ. In Dr. Utz' series, factors predicted for an
unfavorable outcome of patients with ca-in-situ were the
following:
1) Persistent bladder symptomatology.
2) Urinary cytology which has not reverted to normal
   within 6 months after conservative therapy.
3) The presence of ca-in-situ in the urethra, or
   persistent severe irritative bladder symptoms.

This spectrum of abnormalities was associated with invasion in
a substantial proportion of patients and, hence, raises the
possibility of considering earlier cystectomy in this group of
high-risk individuals.


SUGGESTED REFERENCES

General

1. Soloway, M.S.: Rationale for intensive intravesical
   chemotherapy for superficial bladder cancer. J. Urol.
   123:461, 1980.

2. Soloway, M.S.: The management of superficial bladder
   cancer. Cancer 45:1856, 1980.

3. Utz, D.C. and DeWeerd, J.H.: The management of low grade,
   low stage carcinoma of the bladder. In: Skinner, D.G.,
   deKernion, J.B., eds.: Genitourinary Cancer. Philadelphia,
   W.B. Saunders Company, pp. 256, 1978.

4. Heney, N.M. et al. (NBCC Group A): Superficial bladder
   cancer: Progression and recurrence. Proc. Amer. Urol.
   Assoc, 1981 Annual Meeting, Boston, MA; p. 228 (545)
   (Abstract).

Thiotepa

5. Robinson, M.R.G., et al. Intravesical epodyl in the
   management of bladder tumors: Combined experience of the
   Yorkshire urological cancer research group. J. Urol.
   117:972, 1977.

6.  Nieh, P.T., et al.: The effect of intravesical thiotepa on normal and tumor urothelium. J. Urol. 119:59, 1978.

7.  Nocks, B.N., Nieh, P.T. and Prout, G.R., Jr.: A longitudinal study of patients with superficial bladder carcinoma successfully treated with weekly intravesical thio tepa. J. Urol. 122:27, 1979.

Adriamycin

8.  Garnick, M.B., et al.: The treatment of recurrent superficial bladder carcinoma with intravesical adriamycin. Proc. Amer. Soc. Clin. Oncol. 22:109, 1982 (Abstract).

9.  Garnick, M.B., et al.: Clinical pharmacologic evaluation of intravesical adriamycin for recurrent superficial bladder carcinoma. Proc. Amer. Urol. Assoc. 1982 Annual Meeting, Kansas City, MO; p. 189 (445) (Abstract).

10. Bankes, M.D., et al.: Topical instillation of doxorubicin hydrochloride in the treatment of recurring superficial transitional cell carcinoma of the bladder. J. Urol. 118:757, 1977.

11. Mishina, T., et al.: Adriamycin instillation therapy for bladder tumors. Tohoku J. Exp. Med. 127:339, 1979.

Mitomycin-C

12. DeFuria, M.D., et al.: Phase I-II study of Mitomycin C topical therapy for low-grade, low-stage transitional cell carcinoma of the bladder: An interim report. Cancer Treat. Rep. 64:225, 1980.

13. Lockhart, J.L., et al.: Prostatic transitional cell carcinoma after treatment of recurrent superficial bladder tumors with Mitomycin C. Proc. Amer. Urol. Assoc. 1982 Annual Meeting, Kansas City, MO; p. 189 (448) (Abstract).

BCG

14. Lamm, D.L., Stogdill, V.D. and Thor, D.E.: BCG immunotherapy in superficial transitional cell carcinoma of the urinary bladder. Proc Amer. Soc Clin. Oncol. 21:372, 1980 (Abstract).

Carcinoma-in-situ

15. Utz, D.C., et al.: Carcinoma in situ of the bladder.
    Cancer 45:1842, 1980.

16. Utz, D.C., et al.: Experience with cystectomy as primary
    treatment for in situ cancer of the bladder. Proc. Amer.
    Urol. Assoc. 1982 Annual Meeting, Kansas City, MO; p. 188
    (442) (Abstract).

17. Prout, G.R., et al.: The results of conservative treatment
    in patients with carcinoma in situ of the bladder. Proc.
    Amer. Urol. Assoc. 1982 Annual Meeting, Kansas City, MO;
    p. 183 (424) (Abstract).

CHAPTER 14

THE ROLE OF SURGERY IN THE MANAGEMENT OF INVASIVE BLADDER
CANCER


Jerome P. Richie and Donald G. Skinner



Carcinoma of the bladder represents a spectrum of clinical
pathologic entities that find expression in a variety of
biological potential. The assessment and management of
patients with bladder cancer, especially those with tumors
that invade beyond the lamina propria (stage B or greater),
represent a formidable challenge to the urologist, radiotherapist, and medical oncologist. The natural history of bladder
tumors is such that a subset of patients will evidence new
growths in various portions of the bladder, usually of the
low-stage and low-grade variety. The majority of these tumors
can be treated  satisfactorily by transurethral resection, and
rapidly recurring tumors may be treated by intravesical chemotherapy (see Chapter 13). Although the majority of patients
with low-grade and low-stage tumors will continue to have
local recurrences only, a defined population will progress to
more advanced (invasive) disease and require more radical
procedures to effect "cure."

Bladder tumors may be defined in a variety of ways, but
the pathological features of histologic grade and clinical
stage seem to be two of the most important factors. Tumor
stage represents the best indication of the malignant potential of the bladder neoplasm and, as such, is the most relevant factor related to aggressive treatment and subsequent
prognosis. The multicentricity of tumor recurrence in space
and time represents another important factor in the decision
for aggressive therapy. The presence of carcinoma in situ, a
high-grade, non-papillary involvement of the epithelial surface, usually in an area without obvious cystoscopic change,

109

represents an important expression of malignant potential that
should directly influence the need for more aggressive
therapy. Tumor grade is also regarded as an indication of
growth potential, as represented by the fact that  most high-
grade tumors are deeply infiltrating and the incidence of
understaging in high-grade tumors is substantial.

Appropriate assessment of the patient and the state of his
tumor should precede treatment. Assessment includes the overall evalutation of the patient's physical health and emotional status to tolerate the proposed therapy, clinical
staging to select the best therapy to control the tumor and
preserve function, and involvement of appropriate family
members for support and followup care. Clinical staging gives
a histologic diagnosis of the grade and stage of the tumor,
and bimanual examination complements the transurethral resection. Additional staging studies should include chest x-ray,
liver function tests, and bone scan.

Considerations in the therapeutic management of invasive
bladder cancer should include the possibility of surgery,
irradiation, or both. Radiation therapy alone has proven
unsatisfactory in the therapy of deeply infiltrating bladder
tumors. Furthermore, there is no evidence that radiation
therapy prevents the formation of new tumors. Radical cystectomy, to include the prostate, seminal vesicles, and bladder
with surrounding perivesical tissue, as well as the regional
lymph nodes, has been reasonably successful in controlling
local disease in the male patient with infiltrating carcinoma
of the bladder. In females, the operative procedure should
include the uterus, tubes, ovaries, and an anterior cuff of
the vagina as well as the regional lymph nodes.

The indications for radical cystectomy include: 1) Low
stage tumors unsuitable for TUR because of multicentricity,
rapid recurrrences, or high grade lesions. 2) High stage
tumors with evidence of invasion into the muscular layer, even
superficially into the muscle wall. 3) Low grade tumors with
associated carcinoma in situ that have not responded to
intravesical chemotherapy.

Segmental resection has been advocated by some urologists
as an effective procedure to remove the bladder cancer without
altering the normal dynamics of micturition. However, one
must be cognizant that segmental resection is rarely indicated
in primary urothelial tumors. Stringent criteria must be fol-

lowed in an attempt to prevent tumor recurrence or spillage.
The tumor must be unifocal, well away from the ureteral ori-
fices or the bladder neck (at least a 2 cm. margin), and there
must be no evidence of carcinoma in situ or significant atypia
on cold cup random biopsies. Furthermore, prior to a procedure that has the potential to spill bladder tumor cells outside of the bladder, preoperative radiation therapy of at
least 1000 rads should be utilized. Van der Werf-Messing has
clearly shown that a small amount of radiation therapy will
prevent local wound seeding, especially in patients with high
grade carcinoma of the bladder. In the Mayo Clinic series of
3400 patients with bladder cancer, only 199 fit the rigid
criteria for partial cystectomy. Thus, with proper selection,
this operation should rarely be indicated.

Pelvic lymph node metastases have been documented to occur
in 10-50% of patients, the involvement increasing with increasing stage of the primary tumor. Pelvic lymphadenectomy
with removal of micrometastases has led to 5-year survivals of
18-33%. Thus, there may be some therapeutic role for pelvic
lymphadenectomy as well as a prognostic one. It would appear
from the M.D. Anderson series that full field pelvic radiotherapy of 5000 rads over a 5 week period can control microscopic metastases. We feel that the lymphadenectomy allows a
lower dose of radiation therapy to be given, aids in defining
the vascular pedicles of the bladder, provides important
staging information for adjuvant therapy, and adds little to
the operating time or morbidity of the procedure. Therefore,
we recommend pelvic lymphadenectomy in conjunction with
radical cystectomy.

Radical cystectomy has been utilized as the major therapeutic procedure for carcinoma of the bladder, as a salvage
procedure after failure of radiation therapy, or in conjunction with planned preoperative radiation therapy. A single
stage procedure seems more efficacious than a 2-stage procedure, which has not been shown to lower morbidity or mortality
and which has the disadvantage of increased cost, two hospi-
talizations, and two separate anesthetics.

Radiotherapy alone has been conclusively shown to be
inferior to combined therapy with preoperative irradiation and
radical cystectomy. In the M.D. Anderson series, Miller and
Johnson reported 46% five-year survival for patients treated
with preoperative radiotherapy and cystectomy, as opposed to a
16% survival for patients with definitive radiotherapy

alone. Wallace and Bloom reported on 189 patients randomized
to receive 6000 rad radiation therapy or 4000 rad radiation
followed by radical cystectomy 4 weeks later. In this randomized series, the 5-year survival rate was 21% for radiotherapy
alone and 33% for radiotherapy plus radical cystectomy.

Radiotherapy alone can render the bladder free of tumor in
approximately 30% of patients, but the possibility of later
recurrence and the need for "salvage" cystectomy, as well as
limitations to further chemotherapy or increase in difficulty
of surgical procedures, detracts from the alternative of radiation therapy as primary treatment. However, its role as a
preoperative adjunct to cystectomy continues to be touted by
many authors. Logical arguments supporting the use of preoperative radiation therapy include its effect against locally
extensive invasive cancers, its prevention of seeding or subsequent distant metastases, and its control of the tumor
locally.

There is no question that preoperative radiation therapy
and cystectomy today is superior to cystectomy alone 20 years
ago. However, in the past decade there has been an appreci-
able drop in the operative mortality rate and improvement in
the accuracy of staging. The evidence to date is not as
strong to support the superiority of combined radiotherapy
plus cystectomy over cystectomy alone in 1982. The only
clinical trial which has addressed this question is that of
the National Surgical Adjuvant Bladder Project, which compared
radical cystectomy alone to preoperative radiation therapy
plus radical cystectomy. The only statistically significant
advantage to radiation therapy was in those patients who were
downstaged to $P_0$. If one compares the 5-year survival
results of patients with clinical stage B and C tumors, 37% of
those who received combination therapy survived 5 years compared to 29% of those who received definitive surgery alone.

An additional area of controversy concerns the dosage of
preoperative radiotherapy to be utilized. Many patients have
received 4000-5000 rads over a 4-5 week period, with a 4 week
hiatus prior to cystectomy. Whitmore and Skinner and Kaufman
have reported good results with short-course high-dose frac-
tionation, 1600-2000 rad over 4-5 days, followed by immediate
radical cystectomy and pelvic lymphadenectomy. The results of
these series are comparable to those of the longer course of
radiation therapy.

   Skinner and Lieskovsky have recently reviewed their
10-year experience with approximately 200 patients treated by
radical cystectomy. The first 100 were treated with planned
preoperative radiation therapy of 2000 rad over 5 days followed by immediate cystectomy. The second 100 patients were
treated without preoperative radiation therapy. The relative
distribution of clinical stage is equal in the 2 groups. The
actuarial 5-year survival for the 2 groups is virtually identical. Thus, it may be possible that cystectomy alone in 1982
is as efficacious as combined radiation therapy and radical
cystectomy. Prospective randomized studies, planned by the
National Bladder Collaborative Group, should answer this
question definitively.

   In any event, the results of therapy for invasive carcinoma of the bladder are poor under the best of circumstances.
At least 40% of patients develop recurrent disease, 2/3 of
which are in distant sites with or without local pelvic recurrence. No treatment program directed strictly to the pelvis
can hope to improve substantially cure rates unless therapy is
instituted earlier or unless effective systemic chemotherapy
or immunotherapy is added to the therapeutic regimen. One
approach that may be considered is earlier aggressive therapy
in patients in whom the natural history may be predicted
accurately enough to identify those whose tumors will become
invasive and potentially lethal. The red cell adherence test,
associated carcinoma in situ, chromosomal analysis, and tests
that are being newly developed may aid in the identification
of the high-risk patient.

   With improved techniques of preoperative digitalization,
adequate hydration, careful intraoperative monitoring, and
postoperative anticoagulation, the mortality rate for radical
cystectomy and urinary conduit diversion has been reduced to
less than 1%. This very acceptable mortality rate, and low
morbidity rate, would favor the institution of radical
cystectomy at an earlier point in patients at high risk of
metastases and potentially lethal disease.


SELECTED REFERENCES

1.   Johnson, D.E. and Lamy, S.M.:  Complications of
     single-stage radical cystectomy and ileal conduit
     diversion:  Review of 124 cases.  J. Urol.  117:171,
     1977.

2.  Dretler, S.P., Ragsdale, B.D. and Leadbetter, W.F.: The
    value of pelvic lymphadenectomy in the surgical treatment
    of bladder cancer. J. Urol. 109:414, 1973.

3.  Prout, G.R., Jr.: The role of surgery in the potentially
    curative treatment of bladder cancer. Cancer Res.
    37:2764, 1977.

4.  Skinner, D.G.: Current perspectives in the management of
    high-grade invasive bladder cancer. Cancer 45:1866, 1980.

5.  Althausen, A.F., Prout, G.R., Jr. and Daly, J.J. :
    Non-invasive papillary carcinoma of the bladder associated
    with carcinoma in situ. J. Urol. 116:575, 1976.

6.  Richie, J.P., Skinner, D.G. and Kaufman, J.J.: Radical
    cystectomy for carcinoma of the bladder: Sixteen years'
    experience. J. Urol. 113:186, 1975.

7.  Miller, L.S.: Bladder cancer: Superiority of
    preoperative irradiation and cystectomy in clinical stages
    $B_2$ and C. Cancer 39:973, 1977.

8.  Wallace, D.M. and Bloom, H.J.G.: The management of deeply
    infiltrating ($T_3$) bladder carcinoma: Controlled trial
    of radical radiotherapy versus preoperative radiotherapy
    and radical cystectomy (first report). Brit. J. Urol.
    48:587, 1976.

9.  Van der Werf-Messing, B.: Carcinoma of the bladder
    $T_3N_xM_0$ treated by preoperative irradiation therapy
    followed by cystectomy. Cancer 36:718, 1975.

10. Whitmore, W.F., Jr., et al.: A comparative study of two
    preoperative radiation regimens with bladder cancer.
    Cancer 40:1077, 1977.

11. Utz, D.C., Hanash, K.A. and Farrow, G.M.: The plight of
    the patient with carcinoma in situ of the bladder. J.
    Urol. 103:160, 1970.

CHAPTER 15

RADIATION THERAPY IN THE MANAGEMENT OF BLADDER CANCER

Samuel Hellman


The goal in treatment of any tumor is to eradicate the disease locally and regionally and to prevent distant metastases without deleteriously affecting function or structure. Bladder cancer offers difficulty in achieving these goals. The difficulty in local control by either surgery or radiation is manifest by disturbingly high local recurrence figures. There are no good regional treatments for grossly involved lymph nodes or extensive involvement of perivesical structures. There is no curative treatment for already widely disseminated bladder cancer. The morbidity of treatment appears to be significant, and this must be weighed against the gains of treatment. Loss of the bladder, impotence, incontinence, continued dysuria, hematuria, rectal bleeding, and diarrhea may all be complications of the surgical or radiotherapeutic treatment of bladder cancer. Survival alone is not a satisfactory endpoint when the morbidity produced by treatment is extensive.

In this presentation I shall consider the effects of radiation in the treatment of bladder cancer as definitive treatment and as adjuvant treatment either preoperatively or postoperatively.


DEFINITIVE RADIATION THERAPY FOR BLADDER CANCER

There are reports in the literature of supervoltage radiation used in the treatment of bladder cancer of a variety of different stages. Clinical stage $B_2$ and C treated by radiation have been reported by a number of groups with survival rates of approximately 30% with 40-50% local failures. These

data are difficult to evaluate since patients of many stages
are lumped together.  It does appear, however, that when these
results are compared with surgery, there is a 10-15% advantage
to cystectomy as compared to primary radiation therapy.  This
must be modified since some radiation therapy failure patients
can be salvaged with subsequent cystectomy.  Unfortunately the
majority of patients with bladder cancer with significant
muscle invasion die of their disease.  For those patients who
would die of their disease regardless of treatment, clearly
radiation therapy is less toxic and to be preferred.  For
those who will survive with their disease if treated with
either radiation or surgery then radiation is the desired
treatment.  It is only for that group (10-15%) for whom
radiation is not satisfactory treatment that cystectomy is to
be preferred.  The size of this group as compared to the
others must be compared to the morbidity imposed upon the
group at large.

The morbidity of definitive radiation therapy using
external beam techniques can be minimized using modern radiotherapeutic approaches of careful evaluation of tumor location, treatment, simulation, beam localization and treatment.
If the patient has a reasonable bladder capacity at the onset
(without extensive previous fulguration) then good bladder
function after treatment is the rule.  Potency can be pre-
served in approximately 50% of these patients, and rectal
complications may be quite infrequent.  Occasional hematuria
does occur but this is rarely a significant problem.

In patients with early superficial bladder cancer, widespread or recurring frequently following fulguration, radiation may play a useful role.  These patients may be treated
with external beam limited to include only the bladder rather
than the bladder and regional lymph nodes.  Such limitation of
treatment markedly reduces the acute and late complications of
irradiation.  Often such treatment can be combined with intravesical instillation of sealed radioactive sources.  Use of a
central source of radioactivity carefully placed in the bladder may uniformly irradiate the bladder mucosa without excessive dose to more distant tissues.  This should not be used
alone but can be served as a way of boosting the bladder
mucosal dose.

A most exciting approach to localized (less than 5 cm.)
invasive bladder cancer $T_1$ - $T_3$ has been the use of radium
needle implantation technique.  Van der Werf-Messing has
reported 5-year survival figures for $T_1$, $T_2$ and $T_3$
lesions which are remarkably good.  Further she has indicated
that scar recurrences can be markedly reduced with 350 rads x

3. She follows this with a radium needle implant placed
through a suprapubic incision. Bloom and Wallace also
reported a smaller series with similar results. This technique appears to offer promise in the treatment of localized
bladder cancer even with muscle invasion.


ADJUVANT RADIATION THERAPY

     Radiation therapy can be used preoperatively or post-
operatively in combination with cystectomy in order to improve
local and regional control. The rational for pre operative
irradiation is that such treatment will reduce seeding occur-
ing locally or distantly due to manipulation of the tumor at
the time of surgery. It will also be useful for the destruc-
tion of subclinical disease in the bladder, perivesical
structures or the regional lymph nodes. There have been a
number of reports of such treatment and a randomized study
appears to show a difference in survival although this difference did not reach statistical significance. There was,
however, a statistically significant difference in the probability of local control. Forty eight percent of those
patients treated with cystectomy alone in the randomized trial
developed local recurrence.
     The dose of radiation necessary in preoperative irradia-
tion is uncertain. There are two purposes for such treatment,
and one must consider each separately when determining dose.
For the prevention of seeding, it appears from Van der Werf-
Messing's data, as well as others, that quite a low dose of
radiation may be effective. A dose of 1050 rads in 3 days
appears quite satisfactory. The treatment of subclinical
disease in lymph nodes and perivesical structures requires a
greater dose of radiation. In order for this to be given
without excessive toxicity, the fraction size should probably
be kept quite small. While the doses used vary, most radio-
therapists prefer at least 4000-5000 rads given in fraction
sizes of approximately 200 rads per day. Some accelerated
schedules have been used both by us and others; their results
need to be evaluated before they can be accepted.
     Radiation may also be used postoperatively, with the
advantage of avoiding unnecessary irradiation. Those patients
found at surgery to have widespread disease and not suitable
for cystectomy can have their tumors properly mapped and
evaluated and appropriate palliative plan made. This may
include radiation for local control. Those patients who have
only superficial tumors without evidence of extension may not

require radiation. The disadvantages of postoperative radiation appear to be that the morbidity is greater due to fixed loops of bowel in the target area. Tumor control may not be as effective. Some tumor cells may have seeded outside the field, and tumor cells left behind may be rendered somewhat hypoxic and thus less sensitive to radiation. The data reported for such postoperative treatment appear to indicate that the treatment is less efficacious than preoperative treatment, and we do not recommend this routinely.

There is an exciting new possibility for the use of intraoperative radiation therapy, either alone or in combination with external beam. The tumor can be treated by electron beam irradiation or orthovoltage irradiation in the operating room through a suprapubic incision. Careful beam selection and localization can avoid damage to most of the normal tissues. An initial experience by Matsumoto using a single electron beam treatment of 3000 rads indicated a very low incidence of local recurrence.

SUGGESTED REFERENCES

1.  Blandy, J.P. et al.: T3 Bladder Cancer--The case for salvage cystectomy. Brit. J. Urol. 52:506, 1980.

2.  Caldwell, W.L.: The role of irradiation in the management of clinical stage B1 (Grades II and III) and stages B2 and C bladder cancer. Cancer Res. 37:2759, 1977.

3.  Crawford, E.D. and Skinner, D.G.: Salvage cystectomy after irradiation failure. J. Urol. 123:32, 1980.

4.  Cummings, K.B., et al.: Current concepts in the management of patients with deeply invasive bladder carcinoma. Sem. Oncol. 6:220, 1979.

5.  DeWeerd, J.H. and Colby, M.Y., Jr.: Bladder carcinoma treated by irradiation and surgery: interval report. J. Urol. 109:409, 1973.

6.  Goffinet, D.R., et al.: Bladder cancer: results of radiation therapy in 384 patients. Rad. 117:149, 1975.

7.  Goodman, G.B., et al.: Conservation of bladder function in patients with invasive bladder cancer treated by definitive irradiation and selective cystectomy. Int. J.

Radiat. Oncol. 7:559, 1981.

8.  Matsumoto, L., et al.: Clinical evaluation of
    intraoperative radiotherapy for carcinoma of the urinary,
    bladder. Cancer, In Press, 1983.

9.  Miller, L.S.: Bladder cancer. Superiority of preoperative
    irradiation therapy and cystectomy in clinical stages B2
    and C. Cancer 39:973, 1977.

10. Miller, L.S. and Johnson, D.E.: Megavoltage radiation for
    bladder carcinoma: Alone, postoperative, or pre-operative.
    Seventh National Cancer Conference Proceedings, 771, 1973.

11. Mohiuddin, M., et al.: Combined pre- and post-operative
    adjuvant radiation therapy for bladder cancer. Results of
    RTOG-Jefferson study. Cancer 47:2840, 1981.

12. Prout, G.R., Jr., Slack, N.H. and Bross, I.J.:
    Preoperative irradiation as an adjuvant in the management
    of invasive bladder carcinoma. J. Urol. 105:223, 1971.

13. Shipley, W.U.: Radiation therapy for patients with bladder
    carcinoma:  Rationale, results, techniques and possible
    innovations. AUA Monographs, Vol. 1, Chapter 19:243, 1979.

14. Slack, N.H., Bross, I.J. and Prout, G.R., Jr.: Five year
    follow-up results of a collaborative study of therapies
    for carcinoma of the bladder. J. Surg. Oncol. 9:393, 1977.

15. Van der Werf Messing, B.: Cancer of the urinary bladder
    treated by interstitial radium implant. Int. J. Radiat.
    Oncol. 4:373, 1978.

16. Van der Werf Messing, B.: Preoperative radiation followed
    by cystectomy to treat carcinoma of the urinary bladder.
    Int. J. Radiat. Oncol. 5:394, 1979.

17. Van der Werf Messing, B., Star, W.M. and Memon, R.S.:
    T3NXMO bladder cancer treated by radium implant and
    external irradiation. Int. J. Radiat. Oncol. 6: 1723,
    1980.

18. Wallace, D.N. and Bloom, H.J.G.: The management of deeply
    infiltrated bladder carcinoma: Control trial of radical
    radiotherapy vs. pre-operative radiotherapy in radical

cystectomy. Brit. J. Urol. 48:587, 1976.

19. Whitmore, W.F., Jr.,: Combined radiotherapy and surgical treatment of patients with bladder carcinoma. JAMA 207:349, 1969.

20. Whitmore, W.F., Jr., et al.: A comparative study of two preoperative radiation regimens with cystectomy for bladder cancer. Cancer 40:1077, 1977.

CHAPTER 16

SYSTEMIC CHEMOTHERAPY IN THE MANAGEMENT OF BLADDER CANCER

Lawrence H. Einhorn

I. INTRODUCTION

A. 36,000 cases; 10,300 deaths

B. Staging workup - for proven metastatic disease
   1. History & physical
   2. CBC, SMA
   3. CEA
   4. PA & Lateral Chest X-ray
   5. Bone Scan
   6. Abdominal CT (if appropriate)

II. SINGLE AGENT CHEMOTHERAPY

A. Platinum most active drug; no evidence of superiority for Platinum combination chemotherapy vs. single agent Platinum.

B. Methotrexate probably has a similar degree of activity but shorter duration of remission.

C. Other single agents with 10-20% response rates include:
   1. Adriamycin
   2. 5-FU
   3. Cyclophosphamide
   4. Vinblastine
   5. Mitomycin-C

D.  Hexamethylmelamine is the most active agent for
    schistosomiasis-induced Egyptian bladder cancer
    (4); however, same dosage of hexamethylmelamine
    failed to demonstrate therapeutic efficacy in
    transitional cell carcinoma of the bladder in the
    United States.

E.  PHASE II DRUGS
    1.  AMSA - inactive
    2.  Mitoxantrone - inactive
    3.  VP-16 - less than 20% response rate
    4.  VM-26 - less than 20% response rate
    5.  Neocarzinostatin - inactive

III.  NON-PLATINUM COMBINATION CHEMOTHERAPY

A.  Cyclophosphamide + Adriamycin + 5-FU (CAF) vs.
    single agent 5-FU - 3 of 21 responses (14%) for CAF
    vs. 4 of 18 (22%) for 5-FU.

B.  Methotrexate + Adriamycin + Cyclophosphamide (14) -
    2 C.R. and 8 P.R. in 26 patients (38%) with median
    duration of remission 7 months.

C.  Adriamycin + 5-FU
    1.  Wayne State - 8 of 21 (38%) responses
    2.  E.O.R.T.C. - 21 of 52 (40%) responses

IV.  SINGLE AGENT PLATINUM

    1.  Most widely studied agent
    2.  Response rate approximately 40% in patients with no
        prior chemotherapy, with a median duration of 6
        months.
    3.  Complete remissions rare
    4.  More recent studies, including bladder tumor study
        group protocol, suggest response rate may be closer
        to 20%.

V.  PLATINUM COMBINATION CHEMOTHERAPY

A.  Memorial experience (Dr. Yagoda)
    1.  Platinum alone - 10 of 22 (45%) response rate

in patients with no prior chemotherapy.
2. Platinum + Cyclophosphamide - 15 of 32 (47%).
3. Platinum + Adriamycin - 14 of 28 (50%).
4. Platinum + Cyclophosphamide + Adriamycin - 14 of 29 (48%)

B. Indiana University - Platinum + Adriamycin + 5-FU
1. 18 of 39 responses (46%)
2. Median duration response 6 months
3. Median survival for all patients 9 months

C. M.D. Anderson - "CISCA"
1. Initial response rate 90% (9 of 10 patients).
2. However, updated results reveal only 17 of 41 (41%) responses.


VI. PLATINUM RANDOMIZED STUDIES

A. SWOG - Adriamycin vs. Adriamycin + Platinum
1. 20% vs. 41% response rate, but no difference in survival.

B. ECOG - Platinum vs. Cyclophosphamide + Adriamycin + Platinum
1. 24% vs. 37% response rates in 80 patients (not statistically significantly different).
2. 44% of patients with no prior chemotherapy responded.
3. No difference in survival.

C. SECSG - Platinum vs. Cyclophosphamide + Adriamycin + Platinum - results still pending.

D. CALGB - Platinum vs. Cyclophosphamide + Adriamycin + 5-FU - no difference.

E. National Bladder Cancer Collaborative Group A - Platinum vs. Platinum + Cyclophosphamide.
1. 21% response rate (9-43) for Platinum and only 13% (6-47) for combination.

VII.  NEW AVENUES

    A.  New phase II agents
        1.  Tumor stem cell assay (See Chapter 29)

    B.  Platinum analogues

    C.  Better Platinum combinations, e.g., Platinum +
        Methotrexate.

    D.  Adjuvant chemotherapy in invasive bladder cancer.


SUGGESTED REFERENCES

1.  Turner, A.G., et al.: The treatment of advanced bladder
    cancer with Methotrexate. Brit. J. Urol. 49:673, 1977.

2.  Yagoda, A.: Methotrexate in bladder cancer. Proc. Amer.
    Soc. Clin. Oncol. 21:427, 1980 (Abstract).

3.  Blumenreich, et al.: Phase II trial of vinblastine sulfate
    in transitional cell carcinoma. Proc. Amer. Soc. Clin.
    Oncol. 22:466, 1981 (Abstract).

4.  Gad-el Mawla, N.M., et al.: Chemotherapeutic management of
    carcinoma of the bilharzial bladder: A phase II trial with
    Hexamethylmelamine and VM-26.  Cancer Treat. Rep. 62:993,
    1978.

5.  Martino, S., et al.: Phase II study of 5-FU and Adriamycin
    in transitional cell carcinoma of the urinary tract.
    Cancer Treat. Rep. 64:161, 1980.

6.  EORTC Urological Group B: The treatment of advanced
    carcinoma of the bladder with a combination of adriamycin
    and 5-FU. Eur. Urol. 3:276, 1977.

7.  Yagoda, A., et al.: Cis-diamminedichloroplatinum in
    advanced bladder cancer. Cancer Treat. Rep. 60:917, 1976.

8.  Yagoda, A., et al.: Cis-platinum regimens in bladder
    cancer. Proc. Amer. Soc. Clin. Oncol. 20:397, 1979.
    (Abstract).

9.  Williams, S.D., Einhorn, L.H., and Donohue, J.P.:

Cis-platinum combination chemotherapy of bladder cancer. Cancer Clin. Trials 2:335, 1979.

10. Sternberg, J.J., et al.: CISCA for advanced urinary tract carcinoma. JAMA 238:2282, 1977.

11. Gagliano, R.: Adriamycin vs. Adriamycin + cis-platinum in transitional cell carcinoma. A SWOG study. Proc. Amer. Soc. Clin. Oncol. 21:347, 1980 (Abstract).

12. Khandekar, J.D., et al.: Comparative activity and toxicity of platinum in disseminated transitional cell carcinoma of the urinary tract. Proc. Amer. Soc. Clin. Oncol. 22:461, 1981 (Abstract).

13. Einstein, A., et al.: Platinum vs. Platinum + Cyclophosphamide for metastatic bladder cancer. Proc. Amer. Soc. Clin. Oncol. 22:461, 1981 (Abstract).

14. Tannock, I., et al.: Methotrexate, Adriamycin, and cyclophosphamide chemotherapy for transitional cell carcinoma of the urinary tract. Proc. Amer. Soc. Clin. Oncol. 22:461, 1981 (Abstact).

CHAPTER 17

RHABDOMYOSARCOMA OF THE BLADDER AND PROSTATE

Alan B. Retik


Rhabdomyosarcoma is the most common soft tissue sarcoma of childhood. Approximately 30% of these tumors affect the genitourinary tract and pelvis of children.

The predilection of rhabdomyosarcoma to the trigone of the bladder, the prostate, the vagina and paratesticular tissues suggests that it arises from mesenchymal cells of the mesonephros. The rhabdomyosarcomas in children are of embryonal cell type consisting of immature mesenchymal cells undergoing variable degrees of differentiation to striated muscle, connective tissue, and possibly smooth muscle. Extensive submucosal growth within a hollow viscus often produces nodular protrusions within the lumen. These protrusions resemble bunches of grapes, leading to the use of the terms sarcoma botryoides. The typical botryoid sarcoma is a polypoid, bulky, grayish, white tumor composed of lobules with occasional hemorrhage; the softness and consistency are proportional to the amount of myxomatous tissue.


STAGING

        We employ the staging classification of Ghavimi.
    Stage I    -Tumor localized, completely resected, regional
               nodes negative
               IA:  Margins clear microscopically
               IB:  Margins not clear microscopically
    Stage II   -Tumor extends to adjacent structures;
               incompletely resected; regional nodes negative.

Stage III  -Tumor extends to adjacent structures;
           incompletely resected; regional nodes positive
Stage IV   -Distant metastases.


RHABDOMYOSARCOMA OF THE BLADDER

The bladder is the most common urologic site of this
neoplasm. The lesion is seen in males more than twice as
frequently as in females. Almost all of the reported cases
have been in children under the age of five years, with the
majority under age three.

These neoplasms grow in such a way that they seldom cause
mucosal ulceration and hematuria until they become very
extensive. The diagnosis is usually made relatively late
because of the age of the patient and his inability to
describe bladder symptoms. Oftentimes, the first sign may be
urinary retention secondary to bladder outlet obstruction. In
a significant number of children, the tumor is palpable supra-
pubically, and in most cases it is initially thought to be a
distended bladder. These tumors are initially locally
invasive, remaining within the superficial tissues and extending down the urethra or, less commonly, into the lower ureter.
Spread to regional nodes and to distal sites occurs relatively
late in the course.

An excretory urogram may demonstrate negative filling
defects usually confined to the lower half of the bladder.
Definitive diagnosis can be made at the time of cystoscopy
with biopsy. On occasion, severe cystitis may mimic the
appearance of this tumor radiologically, and biopsy is
imperative for the diagnosis.


RHABDOMYOSARCOMA OF THE PROSTATE

In rhabdomyosarcoma of the prostate, pain is usually
absent, and the onset of urinary obstruction is insidious.
The tumor may escape detection for a prolonged period of
time. The distended bladder is often palpable and the base of
the bladder is elevated on the excretory urogram. Diagnosis
is confirmed by transurethral biopsy. Prostatic lesions
usually show earlier spread than bladder ones, with local
nodes involved in at least 40% of cases.

TREATMENT

Until relatively recently, radical surgery offered the only
chance for survival. Microscopic involvement of surrounding
organs was common so that cystectomy and a wide excision of
the adjacent structures seemed to offer the only hope of
cure. In spite of radical surgery, long term survival was
confined primarily to patients with stage I disease of the
bladder. Survival with prostatic rhabdomyosarcoma continued
to be rare. The average survival period in these fatal cases
did not exceed one and one-half years with lesions of the
bladder and about eight months with lesions of the prostate.

Combination therapy consisting of surgery, chemotherapy and
radiation began to be extensively used during the 1960's.
Since 1970 the VAC protocol has been employed in treating
children with genitourinary rhabdomyosarcoma. This protocol
consists of a combination of vincristine, Actinomycin-D and
cyclosphosphamide. Chemotherapy is usually continued for two
years and only interrupted if significant leukopenia or
thrombocytopenia occurs. Combination therapy has improved the
survival rate dramatically. The results with a multimodality
therapeutic approach prompted many to question the need for a
mutilating procedure or radical operations in patients with
localized disease. It it now clear that the combination of
radiotherapy, chemotherapy and the body's resources has a
profound effect on microscopic or residual tumor, as it does
in cases of Wilms' Tumor.

In general, total excision of the organ primarily involved
should be done for localized disease. Because occult submucosal extension is the rule with bladder rhabdomyosarcoma,
total cystectomy and urinary diversion is usually deemed
essential. Our two recent cases of rhabdomyosarcoma of the
bladder and prostate had urethral extension, and we feel that
urethrectomy should be employed in both males and females.
The vagina and uterus should be excised if involved. Therefore, with rhabdomyosarcoma of the prostate, cystectomy,
prostatectomy and urethrectomy should be employed in most
instances. We've had one child in whom a radical prostatectomy was performed, and the child has no evidence of
disease six years later. Lymph node resection should be done
routinely.

In our series of nine children with rhabdomyosarcoma of the
bladder or prostate, the five children with Stage I or II

disease are alive, whereas only one of the four children with
Stage III or IV disease has survived. We now feel that early
relatively radical surgery should be performed in children
with Stage I and II pelvic rhabdomyosarcoma along with
chemotherapy and radiation therapy. In stages III and IV
pelvic rhabdomyosarcoma, intensive chemotherapy and radiation
should be the initial treatment with surgery reserved for
patients with residual disease. This multi-therapeutic
approach has dramatically increased the rate of survival.

SUGGESTED REFERENCES

1. Raney, R.B., et al.: Paratesticular rhabdomyosarcoma in
   childhood. Cancer 42:729, 1978.

2. Ghavimi, F., et al.: Multidisciplinary treatment of
   embryonal rhabdomyosarcoma in children. Cancer 35:677,
   1975.

3. Exelby, P.R., Chauimi, F. and Jereb, B.: Genitourinary
   rhabdomyosarcoma in children. J. Ped. Surg. 13:746, 1978.

4. Jaffe, N., et al. Rhabdomyosarcoma in children. Improved
   outlook with a multidisciplinary approach. Amer. J. Surg.
   125:482, 1973.

5. Cromie, W.J., Raney, R.B. and Duckett, J.W.: Paratesticular
   rhabdomyosarcoma in children. J. Urol. 122:80, 1979.

6. Ortega, J.A.: A therapeutic approach to childhood pelvic
   rhabdomyosarcoma without pelvic exenteration. J. Ped.
   94:205, 1979.

7. Dritschilo, A., et al.: The role of radiation therapy in
   the treatment of soft tissue sarcomas of childhood. Cancer
   42:1192, 1978.

SECTION IV


TESTIS CANCER


One of the most exciting areas in cancer medicine over
the past 10-12 years has been the management of patients with
testicular carcinoma.  In great part, the advances represent
improvements in both combination chemotherapy programs, as
well as increased technical skills of urologic oncologists.
The chapters constituting this section give an overview of
chemotherapy programs containing platinum as originally developed at the Indiana University School of Medicine.  The
strategic timing of surgery both in early stages of nonseminomatous disease, as well as the role of surgery following
combination chemotherapy in removing bulky areas of cancer,
are discussed.  The traditional role of radiation therapy in
the management of patients with seminoma concludes this
section.

CHAPTER 18

CHEMOTHERAPY OF TESTIS CANCER

Lawrence H. Einhorn

I.  Introduction

    A. Accounts for only 1% of male malignancy, with
       approximately 5000 new cases per year; however, very
       important disease because:
       1.  Most common carcinoma in 15–35 age group.
       2.  One of few diseases to have serum markers (hCG &
           AFP).
       3.  Fascinating biological disease, e.g.,
           chemotherapy conversion to mature teratoma.
       4.  Highly curable disease.


II. Staging

    A. History & Physical

    B. hCG, AFP, LDH

    C. SMA and CBC

    D. PA and Lateral Chest X-ray; if normal, Whole Lung
       Tomograms

    E. Abdominal C.T. or Ultrasound

    F. Other studies if clinically indicated

III. Historical Perspectives

A. Actinomycin-D and other single agents

B. Vinblastine + Bleomycin

C. Platinum


IV. Platinum + Vinblastine + Bleomycin (PVB)

A. First study 1974-1976 - high dose (0.4 mg/kg)
   vinblastine.
   1. 33/47 (70%) C.R. (complete remissions)
   2. 5/47 (11%) disease free with PVB followed by
      surgical resection.
   3. 28/47 (60%) currently alive and disease-free
      (NED) with minimum followup 6 years.

B. Second study (1976-1978) - randomization to 0.4 vs
   0.3 mg/kg Vinblastine and third arm PVB (0.2 mg/kg
   vinblastine) + Adriamycin.
   1. Reduction of Vinblastine dosage reduced toxicity
      and cure rates were identical in all three arms.
   2. 53/78 (68%) C.R.
   3. 11/78 (14%) disease-free with PVB followed by
      surgical resection.
   4. 58/78 (74%) currently NED with minimum followup 4
      years.

C. Third study (1978-1981) - PVB vs. PVB + Adriamycin;
   after 4 courses (12 weeks), C.R.'s randomized to
   maintenance vinblastine for 20 months vs. no further
   therapy.
   1. Southeastern Cancer Study Group Co-operative
      Study
   2. No difference between PVB and PVB + Adriamycin
   3. Relapse rate not improved with maintenance
      vinblastine -- therefore, only 12 weeks of
      chemotherapy necessary to ensure optimal
      probability of cure.
   4. 113/171 (66%) C.R.
   5. 19/171 (11%) disease free with chemotherapy
      followed by surgical resection.
   6. Relapse rate only 8% -- minimum followup 18
      months.

V.  Surgical Resection of Residual Disease

    A.  Not advised if hCG and/or AFP elevated and patient
        has several anatomical sites of disease.

    B.  if resected specimen reveals necrotic fibrous tissue,
        mature, and/or immature teratoma -- no further
        chemotherapy needed post-operatively.

    C.  If resected specimen reveals persistent carcinoma, 2
        post-op courses of PVB given
        1. This will change the relapse probability from 80%
           (no post-op therapy or post-op vinblastine) to
           20%.

VI.  Salvage Chemotherapy

    A.  Single agent activity of VP-16
        1.  E.O.R.T.C.                6 of 30   responses
        2.  Charing Cross           11 of 24   responses
        3.  Indiana + Vanderbilt     3 of  5   responses
                 Total   20 of 59   (34%)

    B.  Salvage Chemotherapy - for patients who were not
        progressing within 4 weeks of last dosage of platinum
        or bleomycin
               platinum 20 mg/$M^2$ x 5 Q 3 weeks x 4
               VP-16 100 mg/$M^2$ x 5 Q 3 weeks x 4
               Bleomycin* 30 units/week x 12

*Bleomycin deleted if patient not a candidate to receive
further bleomycin.

    C.  Results With Salvage Therapy
             Number of patients:      45
             Complete Remission:      11 (34%)
             NED with chemotherapy
               plus surgery:        13 (29%)
             Total NED:               24 (53%)
             Continuously NED:        17 (38%) range 18-45 mos.
                                   $\bar{c}$ median 36 mos.

SELECTED REFERENCES

1.  Einhorn, L.H. (editor): Testicular Tumors. Masson
    Publishing Co., New York, NY (1980).

2.  Mackenzie, A.R.: Chemotherapy of metastatic testis
    cancer -- Results in 154 patients. Cancer 19:1369, 1966.

3.  Lange, P.H. and Fraley, E.E.: Serum AFP and HCG in
    testis cancer. Urol. Clin. N. Amer. 4:393, 1977.

4.  Samuels, M.L., et al.: Combination chemotherapy in
    germinal cell tumors. Cancer Treat. Rev. 3:185, 1976.

5.  Vugrin, D., et al.: VAB 6 combination chemotherapy in
    the treatment of metastatic testicular tumors. Cancer
    47:833, 1981.

6.  Einhorn, L.H. and Donohue, J.P.: PVB in disseminated
    testicular cancer. Ann. Intern. Med. 87:293, 1977.

7.  Einhorn L.H. and Williams, S.D.: Chemotherapy of
    disseminated testicular cancer. A random prospective
    study. Cancer 46:1339, 1980.

8.  Einhorn, L.H. et al.: The role of maintenance therapy in
    disseminated testicular cancer. New. Engl. J. Med.
    305:727, 1981.

9.  Einhorn, L.H. and Williams, S.D.: Chemotherapy of
    disseminated seminoma. Cancer Clinical Trials 3:307,
    1980.

10. Williams, S.D., et al.: VP-16-213 salvage therapy for
    refractory germinal neoplasms. Cancer 46:2154, 1980.

11. Einhorn, L.H., et al.: Surgical resection in
    disseminated testicular cancer following chemotherapeutic
    cytoreduction. Cancer 48:904, 1981.

CHAPTER 19

THE ROLE OF SURGERY IN EARLY STAGE TESTIS CANCER

Jerome P. Richie and Donald G. Skinner

Testicular cancer, although relatively rare, is the most
frequent malignancy in males between the ages of 20 and 35.
The disease, occurring in a crucial evolutionary period of a
young man's life, carries a profound social, economic, and
emotional impact far beyond its seeming rarity. Delay in
diagnosis is common for a variety of reasons. There are no
early symptoms specific for primary testicular neoplasms other
than slight changes in testicular size and consistency,
usually occurring gradually rather than suddenly. The most
common presenting symptom of a patient with testis tumor is
painless enlargement, occurring in approximately 2/3 of
patients. Other symptoms may include a specific lump, nodule,
or firm induration within the area of testis. Less commonly,
a sensation of a dull ache in the groin may be the only
presenting complaint. Testicular cancer is often confused in
its clinical presentation with acute epididymitis, especially
when the physician sees the patient several days to weeks
after the onset of symptoms. In such a case, testicular
ultrasound is a valuable addition to the physical examination
in order to separate testicular from extra-testicular masses.

Dramatic changes have occurred in the management of
nonseminomatous germ cell tumors of the testis in the past 10
years. Improved chemotherapy has been largely responsible for
enhanced survival, but surgery remains a major factor in the
overall management planning. The role of surgery is three-
fold. First, radical orchiectomy establishes the diagnosis
and should control the primary tumor, regardless of local
tumor growth or histologic pattern. Secondly, a meticulous
thorough retroperitoneal lymph node dissection has consist-

137

ently been the single most important factor in determining
stage of disease and the need for alternate chemotherapy.  In
this country, retroperitoneal lymph node dissection has
totally supplanted the need for radiation therapy in patients
with nonseminomatous testis cancer.  Third, surgery has become
an integral adjuvant to effective platinum-based chemotherapy
in patients with advanced disease.  In patients who do not
achieve complete remission after chemotherapy, retroperitoneal
lymphadenectomy can completely remove massive retroperitoneal
disease.  Furthermore, the histology derived from cytoreductive surgery provides important prognostic information and
direction for the subsequent need for chemotherapy.

Appropriate management of the patient with testicular
tumors is dictated by the primary histology of the tumor and
the clinical stage.  Any patient with suspected tumor of the
testicle should undergo radical orchiectomy.  This is accomplished by an inguinal approach with early mobilization and
clamping of the vessels with a rubber-shod clamp.  The testicle is mobilized into the field and is examined carefully.
If any suspicion of tumor exists, the vessels are ligated and
the specimen removed enbloc.  Transcrotal biopsy is absolutely
contraindicated, as it markedly alters the lymphatic drainage
and recurrence rate, and, hence, overall prognosis.

Evidence that radical orchiectomy controls the primary
tumor may be gleaned from the fact that scrotal recurrence or
subsequent metastasis to the groin is exceedingly rare.  Local
growth pattern, such as invasion of the cord outside the
testis, has no prognostic implications on overall survival, as
long as the testicle is removed via the above-described
approach.

Once the testicle has been removed, careful histological
examination, including step sectioning of the testicle, will
establish the histologic diagnosis.  The most common tumor of
the testicle is seminoma, followed by embryonal carcinoma,
teratoma, and choriocarcinoma.  Combinations of different
types, such as embryonal carcinoma and teratoma (terato-
carcinoma), occur in about 40% of patients.  In our experience, the most important decision is whether the tumor is a
nonseminomatous tumor versus a pure seminoma.  Other than the
extremely rare instance of pure choriocarcinoma (less than 1%
of all nonseminomatous germ cell tumors), experience indicates
that survival is not statistically influenced by cell type of
nonseminomatous testis tumor.

Once the diagnosis of nonseminomatous germ cell tumor has
been established, clinical tests are obtained to ascertain the
stage of tumor. The retroperitoneum is most efficiently evaluated by computed tomography scan, which has largely replaced
intravenous pyelography and/or abdominal ultrasound. Evaluation for other sites of metastatic disease should include
careful palpation of the supraclavicular regions, chest x-ray
and whole lung tomography, and liver function tests. Liver
and bone scans have not been found to be cost effective in the
absence of elevated liver function tests or serum alkaline
phosphatase. Chest film with the lateral view allows for
examination of the mediastinum for possible lymphatic metastases. However, the plain chest film will not identify
pulmonary nodules less than 1 cm in diameter, whereas whole
lung tomography can accurately depict nodules 6 mm in
diameter. The use of CT scan for evaluation of the pulmonary
cavity has not proven to be as effective in identification of
metastases. The CT scan will identify lesions greater than 3
mm in diameter, but many of the smaller lesions represent
non-malignant processes. Thus, we feel that the best accuracy
is gained by the use of lung tomography.

In addition to routine laboratory tests such as complete
blood count, urinalysis, and multichannel analysis, two other
laboratory serum studies (tumor markers) have become of
important value - the beta subunit of human chorionic gonadotropin and alphafetoprotein. These two tumor markers have
improved methods of diagnosis and treatment of testis tumor.
Although the elaboration of human chorionic gonadotropin (hCG)
has been known and measured in the urine for many years, bio-
assays were relatively inefficient and insensitive. The
hormone was easily confused with the cross-reacting lutein-
izing hormone (LH) and, as such, was a relatively insensitive
determination. With the development of a radioimmunossay for
the beta chain of the hCG molecule, this assay can now differ-
entiate reliably between the beta subunit of hCG and the beta
subunit of LH, providing an extremely sensitive method of
identifying small amounts of specific beta-hCG in the serum.
The sensitivity has been increased at least 200 fold.

The second protein tumor marker, alphafetoprotein (AFP),
is produced by the fetal yolk sac and is not present in serum
of individuals after one year of age. A sensitive radioimmunoassay of AFP has allowed detection of this elevated
tumor marker in patients with testicular tumors that would
have been missed by earlier, more insensitive, assays. The

usefulness of these two tumor markers is their sensitivity as an indicator of metastatic disease and their ability to monitor the effectiveness of therapy, predominantly for recurrence.

Alphafetoprotein has never been documented to be elevated in a patient with pure seminoma and, as such, the elevation of this protein in the blood of a patient mandates against the diagnosis of seminoma. Beta hCG may be elevated in approximately 10% of patients with seminoma and has been shown to be elaborated by syncytiotrophoblasts. The elevation of the beta hCG in a patient with the diagnosis of seminoma may indicate nonseminomatous testis tumor or may indicate seminoma with synctiotrophoblastic elements. Whether the seminoma with elevated beta hCG is as responsive to radiation therapy as the garden variety seminoma remains to be elucidated.

Bilateral lymphangiography has not gained universal acceptance as a routine diagnostic procedure. The overall accuracy of lymphangiogram is only 70%, and the sequelae of oil embolization and impairment of pulmonary function may necessitate a delay in planned subsequent surgical therapy. Lymphangiographic dye tends to make the retroperitoneal lymph nodes more reactive, fibrotic, and more difficult to resect, increasing the difficulty of retroperitoneal lymphadenectomy. Furthermore, the reported incidence of false-positive determinations in lymphangiographic studies ranges from 9 to 54 percent with false-negative rates ranging from 9 to 30 percent. Therefore, lymphangiography is not recommended as a routine part of the staging procedure in patients with nonseminomatous testis tumors, as this study has been supplanted by other more effective and less invasive studies.


STAGING

All the tests described are correlated to form a clinical estimate of stage and spread of the testis tumor. The two most commonly utilized systems of staging, proposed by Maier and Skinner, are outlined in Table 19-1 . Accurate staging allows for proper selection of the appropriate form of therapy.

TABLE 19-1. STAGING OF TESTIS TUMORS

| Walter Reed General Hospital | Skinner |
|---|---|
| IA: Confined to testis; no clinical or x-ray evidence of spread | A: Same, but includes no positive nodes on lymph node dissection |
| IB: Same as IA, but at lymph node dissection metastases to iliac or para-aortic lymph nodes | B: Disease below diaphragm, CXR, and mediastinum |
| II: Disease below diaphram/no spread to visceral organs clinical or x-rays evidence of metastases to para-aortic, femoral, inguinal, and iliace lymph nodes. | $B_1$: less than 6 positive nodes that are well encapsulated and no extension to retroperitoneal fat. $B_2$: greater than or equal to 6 positive nodes that are capsular and retroperitoneal fat extension |
| $II^+$: Palpable abdominal mass ( greater than 5 cm) | $B_3$: Bulky abdominal mass ( greater than 5 cm) |
| III: Disease above diaphragm or spread to body organs (clinical x-ray) | C: Metastases above diaphragm. |

In spite of the advanced technology, with the development of CT scan, tumor markers, etc., there are severe limitations to the accuracy of staging. These sophisticated tests are rarely wrong when positive, so that the false-positive rate is quite acceptable. However, a significant false-negative rate exists, especially for the patient with limited nodal involvement in the retroperitoneum.

In regard to clinical staging by means of serum tumor

markers, striking limitations in the sensitivity of currently
available hCG and AFP determinations in the management of
patients without advanced testicular disease are evident.  In
a series of 142 patients with nonseminomatous germ cell
tumors, the incidence of elevated tumor markers, hCG, AFP, or
both, are depicted in Table 19-2.  The incidence of one or
both markers being elevated increases with increasing stage of
disease.  However, 50% of patients with documented stage B-1
testis cancer and 36% of patients with stage B-2 testis cancer
have falsely negative tumor markers.  Thus, tumor markers,
when elevated, depict retroperitoneal or distant involvement;
however, tumor markers, when negative, do not effectively
eliminate the possibility of retroperitoneal nodal involvement.

TABLE 19-2

| STAGE | # PATIENTS | hCG (%) | AFP (%) | EITHER (%) |
|-------|-----------|---------|---------|-----------|
| A     | 67        | 7       | 9       | 10        |
| $B_1$ | 15        | 29      | 33      | 50        |
| $B_2$ | 23        | 52      | 43      | 64        |
| $B_3$ | 6         | 83      | 75      | 100       |
| C     | 31        | 84      | 60      | 93        |

     CT scan, advocated by many as the best test to discern
retroperitoneal nodal involvement, has been reviewed in our
first 30 patients at the Brigham and Women's Hospital.  The
overall accuracy was 70%.  However, the false negative rate,
or reliability of a negative CT scan, was 44%.  This compares
to 37% at the Indiana Hospital and 47% at Memorial Sloan
Kettering Cancer Center.  Thus, a negative CT scan may miss
significant retroperitoneal involvement, even up to 2 to 3 cm
in diameter.

     Lymphangiography, as mentioned above, also has a high
false negative rate, ranging from 37 to 44%.

     All of the above limitations on our clinical ability to
estimate retroperitoneal nodal involvement in patients with
nonseminomatous testis cancer have a profound impact on the
decision for therapy.  There are those individuals who
advocate withholding lymphadenectomy entirely in patients
without evidence of metastases upon presentation, relying upon

improved chemotherapy to salvage those patients that eventually fail.  However, if one contemplates therapy based on
clinical staging with the substantial lack of accuracy shown
above, such patients will be subjected to the need for
extremely close observation.  In addition, such patients will
be subjected to the mental anguish of an unknown prognosis
with many more eventually needing intensive chemotherapy
utilizing drugs with unknown longterm sequelae.  In contrast,
the longterm effects of retroperitoneal lymph node dissection,
with or without less toxic chemotherapy, are well known.


THERAPY

     Controversy exists as to the best form of treatment for
nonseminomatous testis tumors.  The British literature
indicates that radiation therapy has been useful as a primary
modality of treatment.  In the United States, however,
surgical removal of retroperitoneal lymph nodes has been the
mainstay of treatment for clinical low stage testis cancer,
with radiation therapy, chemotherapy, or both reserved as
adjuncts.  Retroperitoneal lymphadenectomy, initially
described in 1902, has developed into an important staging as
well as therapeutic procedure for patients with nonseminomatous testis cancer.  Recently, three major centers have
reported a 97% tumor-free survival for all patients with stage
A and B disease treated since 1973 without exclusion of the
basis of extent of disease.  Basic to the treatment plan at
these centers has been a careful surgical staging by means of
a meticulous retroperitoneal lymph node dissection along with
the subsequent use of adjuvant chemotherapy.  There is now
unequivocal evidence that a meticulous retroperitoneal lymph
node dissection effectively controls local disease with a low
morbidity and a mortality rate of less than 0.5%.  Furthermore, among the 227 collected patients including some with
stage B massive retroperitoneal disease, only 1 retroperitoneal recurrence was documented.  Staubitz, in a series of
patients treated with retroperitoneal lymphadenectomy without
adjunctive radiotherapy or chemotherapy, demonstrated five
year survival rates for stage I and stage II patients of 75%
with retroperitoneal lymphadenectomy alone.  Thus, removal of
the retroperitoneal lymph nodes can be therapeutic as well as
diagnostic.

     Various surgical approaches have been described for extir-
pation of the retroperitoneal lymph nodes in patients with

testis tumors.  The first recorded description of retroperitoneal lymphadenectomy used the transperitoneal approach;
however, the extraperitoneal route became the approach of
choice until the modern era of antibiotics.  Two major approaches are used today, the anterior transabdominal approach
or the extraperitoneal thoracoabdominal approach.

Relative merits of the approaches relate to the primary
testicular lymphatic drainage area, with prevention of the
possibility of contralateral spread of tumor, technical
feasibility of excising lymph nodes, and prevention of
potential complications.  It is worthwhile to recall that the
primary landing site for testicular metastases is located at
L2 on the left and between L1 and L3 on the right, usually
between the aorta and the inferior vena cava.  Crossover
drainage does occur, more frequently from the right side to
the left, but it can occur in either direction.  Because of
this crossover drainage, a bilateral retroperitoneal lymph
node dissection is important.

The question of suprahilar involvement has been an
important one in patients with low-stage testicular cancer.
Donohue has been one of the main advocates of suprahilar
dissection and has clearly detailed the extent of nodal
involvement in a large series of patients with right-sided or
left-sided tumors.  In the patient with very limited microscopic disease, suprahilar nodal involvement is infrequent.
However, in patients with more extensive retroperitoneal nodal
involvement, at least 25% will have suprahilar involvement as
well.  This high number indicates the need for suprahilar
nodal dissection in all but patients without any evidence of
macroscopic disease in the retroperitoneum.

Regardless of which approach is utilized, the operation is
well tolerated in young patients.  The average hospital stay
is 7.2 days, and the operative mortality is less than 0.5%.
There is a low morbidity with the major problem being ejaculatory impotence in approximately 50-70%.  The importance of
ejaculatory impotency, however, may be overstated as many of
these patients have an impairment of contralateral testicular
function with markedly abnormal sperm counts prior to undergoing any retroperitoneal surgery.  Nonetheless, the problem
of ejaculatory impotency is one that has been addressed by
Lange and associates and others.  Impairment of ejaculatory
function occurs either at the level of the sympathetic chain
bilaterally or at the postganglionic sympathetic nerves that

cross over the aortic bifurcation.  Lange and associates have
shown that preservation of ejaculatory capability can be
achieved in at least 50-60% of patients by judicious dissection below the level of the inferior mesenteric artery and the
level of the aortic bifurcation.  In patients with clinical
lack of evidence of macroscopic nodal involvement, this
compromise may be reasonable in an attempt to lessen longterm
morbidity from retroperitoneal lymphadenectomy.

When considering alternate methods of therapy, one must
realize that the results of therapy utilizing a plan of
management based on careful, meticulous surgical staging via
retroperitoneal lymphadenectomy have resulted in the highest
cure rate achieved for any solid tumor in man.  Thus, longterm
comparable data from a large series of patients managed in
another fashion should be available before any major shift in
therapy away from retroperitoneal lymphadenectomy.

Radiation therapy has been utilized to the retroperitoneum
following orchiectomy as a therapy for nonseminomatous tumors
in England.  Tyrell and Peckham reported an 84% two year
disease-free rate for 88 stage A patients and a 58% disease-
free rate for 29 patients with clinical stage B disease.
These survival figures differ considerably from the respective
tumor-free survival rates of 99% for stage A patients and 95%
for stage B patients managed with lymphadenectomy and chemotherapy without radiation.  Furthermore, radiation therapy
makes subsequent use of intensive combination chemotherapy
hazardous, especially the use of platinum-based polychemotherapy.  Several centers in the United States had previously
utilized sandwich irradiation therapy, 2000 rad to the retroperitoneum, followed by retroperitoneal lymphadenectomy,
followed by an additional 2000 rad to the retroperitoneum.  It
is of interest that all of these centers have since abandoned
sandwich irradiation therapy in favor of retroperitonneal
lymphadenectomy, with or without chemotherapy.

With the development of more sensitive tests and perhaps
more sensitive tumor markers to indicate the presence or
absence of retroperitoneal nodal disease, retroperitoneal
lymphadenectomy may have to be reexamined in another light.
However, with the lack of sensitivity of biochemical tumor
markers for minimal disease and our inability to carefully
assess and monitor the retroperitoneal lymph nodes, a
meticulous surgical staging procedure currently allows selection of the least toxic chemotherapeutic agent or combination

tailored to maximize survival of the patient with minimal
morbidity.  By allowing the selection of additional chemotherapy and eliminating retroperitoneal recurrence, retroperitoneal lymphadenectomy remains the single most important
factor in dictating therapeutic plans at the current time.
The tumor-free survival of 97% for all patients with clinical
stage A and B disease represents the gold standard by which
any other therapy must subsequently be compared.

REFERENCES

1.  Donohue, J.P. and Einhorn, L.H.:  Cytoreductive surgery
    for metastatic testis cancer:  Considerations of timing
    and extent.  J. Urol. 123:876, 1980.

2.  Donohue, J.P., Einhorn, L.H. and Perez, J.M.:  Improved
    management of nonseminomatous testis tumors.  Cancer
    42:2903, 1978.

3.  Einhorn, L.H. and Donohue, J:  Cis-diamminedichloro-
    platinum, vinblastine, and bleomycin combination
    chemotherapy in disseminated testicular cancer.  Ann. Int.
    Med. 87:293, 1977.

4.  Garnick, M.B., et al.:  Sequential combination
    chemotherapy and surgery for disseminated testicular
    cancer:  Cis-diamminedichloroplatinum, vinblastine, and
    bleomycin remission induction followed by cyclophosphamide
    and Adriamycin.  Cancer Treat. Rep. 63:1681, 1979.

5.  Hussey, D.H., Luk, K.H. and Johnson, D.E.:  The role of
    radiation therapy in the treatment of germinal cell tumors
    of the testis other than pure seminomas.  Radiology
    123:175, 1977.

6.  Javadpour, N. and Bergman, S.:  Recent advances in
    testicular cancer.  Curr. Prob. Surg. 15:1, 1978.

7.  Lynch, D.F., Jr., et al:  Sandwich therapy in testis
    tumor:  Current experience.  J. Urol. 119:612, 1978.

8.  Richie, J.P.:  Radical retroperitoneal lymphadenectomy for
    testis tumor.  Res. and Staff Phys. 28:50, 1982.

9.  Safer, M.L. et al:  Lymphangiography–accuracy in staging
    of testicular tumor.  Cancer, 35:1603, 1975.

10. Skinner, D.G.:  Nonseminomatous testis tumors:  A plan of
    management based on 96 patients to improve survival in all
    stages by combined therapeutic modalities.  J. Urol.
    115:65, 1976.

11. Skinner, D.G.:  Considerations for management of large
    retroperitoneal tumors:  Use of the modified
    thoracoabdominal approach.  J. Urol.  117:605, 1977.

12. Waters, W.B., Garnick, M.B. and Richie, J.P.:
    Complications of retroperitoneal lymphadenectomy in the
    management of nonseminomatous tumors of the testis.
    Surg., Gynec. & Obstet.  154:501, 1982.

CHAPTER 20

ROLE OF TUMOR REDUCTIVE SURGERY AFTER CHEMOTHERAPY FOR TESTIS
CANCER


Jerome P. Richie


Major advances have been made in the management of testicular cancer in the past 10 years.  Foremost in these advances
has been the discovery of markedly effective combinations of
chemotherapeutic agents that will effect shrinkage of large
solid tumors in the retroperitoneum.  Thus, improvements in
combination chemotherapy have been so impressive that operative therapy and combination chemotherapy now can be combined
effectively to cure the majority of patients with advanced
testicular tumors.  Prior to the discovery of effective
chemotherapy, surgical cytoreduction or debulking was the
primary treatment of choice.  The concept was to reduce tumor
burden so that whatever chemotherapy was available could then
be more effective.

In 1982, however, combination therapy is the primary
treatment of choice for patients with widely metastatic
testicular cancer or large bulky abdominal disease.  Large
volumes of nonseminomatous germ cell tumors of the testis will
seemingly disappear after treatment with combination chemotherapy, especially platinum, vinblastine, and bleomycin.

Although cytoreduction by chemical methods is impressive,
many patients will have evidence of persistent abdominal mass
disease following 4 cycles of platinum-based polychemotherapy.
Furthermore, a reasonable concern has been our lack of specificity and high number of false negative rates for clinical
staging in patients with minimal stage disease.  In a recent
series of 30 patients evaluated by CT scan immediately prior
to retroperitoneal lymphadenectomy, the specificity was 65%
and the false negative rate was 44%.  Thus, a negative CT scan

149

may not exclude retroperitoneal disease. Likewise, tumor
markers, when positive, are highly indicative of metastatic
disease in the retroperitoneum. However, negative tumor
markers have been reported, especially after chemotherapy.
Therefore, a place still exists for tumor reductive surgery
following chemotherapy in patients with residual masses
remaining in the retroperitoneum.

Approximately one-third of patients with persistent
masses after chemotherapy will be found to have viable tumor,
one-third to have only necrosis of fibrosis, and one-third to
have mature teratomatous elements in the contracted tumor
specimen. Operation is required for the effective removal of
the residual mass lesion with the possibility of persistent
cancer as well as for tissue definition. The histology of the
resected specimen further guides the medical oncologist in
decision for additional chemotherapy.


SURGICAL APPROACH

The thoracoabdominal approach is my preferred approach
for patients with large retroperitoneal masses after chemotherapy. Depending upon the predominant side of tumor
involvement, a right or left thoracoabdominal approach is
utilized with incision of the 8th or 7th rib. The incision
should be carried high up in the epigastrium, well above the
umbilicus, and extended downward as a paramedian incision.
The peritoneal cavity should be entered, and the small bowel,
ascending colon, duodenum, and pancreas mobilized by incising
the posterior peritoneum. All of these contents are placed
into a Lahey bag on the anterior abdominal wall. Care must be
taken to protect the superior mesenteric artery. In patients
with left-sided tumor, the descending colonic mesentery may be
divided, carefully protecting the marginal artery. By division of the descending colonic mesentery and freeing of the
lateral surface of the descending colonic peritoneal reflection, the descending colon may be rotated to the left or
right, allowing complete exposure of the residual tumor mass,
great vessels, and ipsilateral kidney. Even extensive mass
lesions can be dissected with this extensive exposure; rarely,
resection of the vena cava or en bloc ipsilateral nephrectomy
is necessitated by the tumor mass.

All of the tissue is divided anterior to the vena cava
and aorta and separated into three packets, 1) lateral to the

aorta, 2) between the aorta and vena cava, and 3) lateral to
the vena cava. The inferior mesenteric artery is routinely
sacrificed, as are all the lumbar arteries and veins from
below the renal hilum.

The importance of a complete retroperitoneal lymphadenectomy cannot be overemphasized. In a recent study by
Donohue and associates, a focus of persistent malignancy was
noted in 37% of patients, often in a small and seemingly
random distribution. The residual cancer was often located
outside of the large bulky residual mass lesion, making biopsy
either intraoperatively or percutaneously inadvisable. Thus,
mere gross examination and biopsy or removal of the central
portion of residual tumor is inadequate because of the varied
nature and distribution of tissue changes after chemotherapy.

Surgical management of a patient who has received extensive amounts of bleomycin requires important and careful
attention to detail. Since patients with bleomycin may have
pulmonary fibrosis, two factors are seemingly important in
reducing the problem of postoperative pulmonary complications. Firstly, these patients are exquisitely sensitive to
the percentage of inspired oxygen. The forced inspiratory
oxygen level should be kept below 25%, and preferably closer
to 20 or 21% throughout the operation and the postoperative
period. Arterial blood gases obtained on room air prior to
the surgical procedure will give an important baseline for the
$pO_2$ in the blood. One additional parameter not to be over-
looked is limited hydration. Increased hydration in the perioperative period increases interstitial edema and, hence, the
requirement for oxygen. Thus, a vicious cycle may be started
requiring higher forced inspiratory oxygen to maintain the
$pO_2$ at acceptable levels. A central venous pressure monitor
should be placed and the patients should be kept at a low CVP
during the perioperative period.

Controversy exists about the management of patients with
stage C disease who have no evidence of retroperitoneal nodal
involvement at the completion of chemotherapy. Initially, our
approach was to explore all such patients. However, we have
found that in patients with clinical complete remission, in
whom no bulky abdominal disease was present initially, the
incidence of residual cancer in the retroperitoneum has been
zero. Accordingly, in patients who achieve a complete
clinical remission by all criteria after multiple dose
chemotherapy, retroperitoneal lymphadenectomy has not been

performed routinely. However, because of the limited ability
of our staging techniques, tumor markers, etc. to delineate
retroperitoneal nodal involvement, these patients require
close observation. We are currently observing our followup
and relapse rates in this group of patients compared to those
who did undergo retroperitoneal lymph node dissection before
definite conclusions can be reached.

The prognosis in patients with residual cancer in the
resected specimen after chemotherapy is variable. In our
series of 54 patients, 7 were found to have residual cancer
after 4 or 5 doses of platinum-based polychemotherapy. Four
of these 7 patients had complete resection of the tumor, and
all 4 are alive without evidence of disease after additional
chemotherapy with cytoxan and adriamycin. In the 3 patients
in whom resection was incomplete, 2 of the 3 are alive with
persistent disease and one has died. Thus, the prognosis in
patients with residual cancer is directly related to the
ability to adequately resect all residual cancer.

Although the surgery for patients with large masses after
chemotherapy is demanding, careful attention to detail can
result in effective cytoreduction and possible cure when
complemented with additional chemotherapy. Operative morbidity and mortality can be kept to a minimum by judicious perioperative management. We conclude that a survival advantage
has been conferred upon patients with bulky abdominal disease
or metastatic disease by the use of combination chemotherapy
followed by appropriate retroperitoneal lymph node dissection
to aid in tissue diagnosis and further therapy. This modality
is particularly important in patients with residual mass
lesions after chemotherapy, as many of these patients can be
rendered in clinical complete remission by the addition of
cytoreductive surgery.

Accelerated growth of non-seminomatous germ cell tumors
has been reported after cytoreductive surgery. However,
analysis of these cases reveals that there was evidence of
active tumor growth at the time of surgical intervention.
These cases represented failure of chemotherapy, and surgical
intervention was utilized as a last means to try to halt the
progress of the tumor. Anesthesia and surgery are suppressors
of the immune response and may allow generalized growth or
enhancement of growth. Therefore, it is imperative that these
patients be under good control with chemotherapy prior to
surgical manipulation.

SUGGESTED REFERENCES

1. Donohue, J.P., Perez, J.M. and Einhorn, L.H.:
   Improved management of non-seminomatous testis
   tumors. J. Urol. 121:425, 1979.

2. Donohue, J.P., Einhorn, L.H. and Williams, S.D.:
   Cytoreductive surgery for metastatic testis cancer:
   Considerations of timing and extent. J. Urol.
   123:876, 1980.

3. Garnick, M.B., et al.: Sequential combination
   chemotherapy in surgery for disseminated testicular
   cancer. Cancer Treat. Rep. 63:1681, 1979.

4. Goldiner, P.L. and Schweizer, O.: The hazards of
   anesthesia and surgery in Bleomycin-treated patients.
   Sem. Oncol. 6:121, 1979.

5. Richie, J.P., Garnick, M.B., and Finberg, H.:
   Computerized Tomography: How accurate for abdominal
   staging of testis tumors? J. Urol. 127:715, 1982.

6. Skinner, D.G.: Non-seminomatous testis tumors: A
   plan of management based on 96 patients to improve
   survival in all stages of combined therapeutic
   modalities. J. Urol. 115:65, 1976.

7. Waters, W.B., Garnick, M.B., and Richie, J.P.:
   Complications of retroperitoneal lymphadenectomy in
   the management of non-seminomatous tumors of the
   testis. Surg. Gynecol. & Obstet. 154:501, 1982.

CHAPTER 21

SEMINOMA

Ralph Weichselbaum

I.  HISTOPATHOLOGY

    A.  Pure Seminoma
        1.  Characterized by polyhedral cells with fine
            definite cytoplasmic membranes, granular or clear
            cytoplasm and centrally placed nuclei with well
            dispersed chromatin.  This is the most common
            form of seminoma.

    B.  Anaplastic Seminoma
        1.  Irregularily clumped chromatin and prominent
            nucleoli characterize this variant.  Giant cells
            are present which may be confused with
            trophoblastic cells.

    C.  Spermatocytic Seminoma
        1.  Cells have round nuclei with coarsly granular and
            dense chromatin.  So named because this variant
            resembles the nuclei of spermatocytes.  It
            comprises 3-8% of all seminomas.


II. RADIOBIOLOGY CONCEPTS

    A.  Seminoma likely dies an intermitotic death, i.e.,
        cell division not requried for the expression of
        cellular lethality.

III. CLINICAL PRESENTATION

   A. Most commonly presents as a scrotal mass. Primary
      differential diagnosis is hydrocele, spermatocele,
      torsion or epidiymitis. Acute pain is uncommon,
      although 30-50% of patients give a history of some
      pain.

   B. History of cryptorchid testis or inguinal or scrotal
      surgery important.


IV. CONFIRMATION OF DIAGNOSIS

   A. Inguinal orchiectomy


V. STAGING PROCEDURES AFTER DIAGNOSIS OF SEMINOMA IS
   ESTABLISHED

   A. PA-lateral roentgenograms

   B. IVP

   C. Pedal lymphangiography

   D. C.T. scan

   E. Serum alpha fetoprotein and beta subunit hCG

   F. Controversial studies
      1. CT scan
      2. Testicular lymphangiogram
      3. Chest tomograms


VI. STAGING SYSTEMS

   A. TMN vs. modified Walter Reed
      1. TMN emphasizes primary tumor size but does not
         utilize biological markers (hCG, AFP) to assess
         disease extent
      2. Most important prognostic factor is involvement
         of retroperitoneum and extent of this
         involvement. IIA includes patients with lesions
         less than 5 cm in diameter and IIB greater than

       5 cm.
    3. Special subset of patients with stage III
       (III$_A$) extension above diaphragm but confined
       to mediastinum and supraclavicular nodes may be
       important.


VII. TREATMENT

   A. Early stage seminoma (I,IIA)
      1. Little disagreement that radiotherapy is the
         mainstay of treatment here. Following orchi-
         ectomy RT is delivered to para-aortic and ipsi-
         lateral pelvic nodes to a dose of 2500-3000 rad
         in 3 weeks. If a scrotal incision was performed,
         this is included in the treatment field with the
         inguinal lymphatics.
      2. Mediastinal treatment. Little data to suggest
         treatment of the mediastinum improves prognosis
         for stage I disease. If it is positive but nodes
         are less than 3 cm (II$_A$), controversy has
         arisen over prophylactic treatment of the
         mediastinum and supraclavicular nodes. Princess
         Margaret Hospital (PMH) claims excellent survival
         in IIA patients without prophylactic treatment.
         Question of salvage addressed below.

   B. Treatment of "Intermediate stage seminoma" (IIB
      greater than 5cm)
      1. Tumor volume plays a large role in the ultimate
         relapse of patients with seminoma. Review of
         literature shows this fact is due to (1) failure
         to include all tumor in irradiated volume and (2)
         the development of extra lymphatic metastasis.
      2. Cure rates with range and masses approximately
         60-65%, 70-75% (PMH, Royal Marsden) depending
         upon tumor size distribution. PMH treats only to
         diaphragm. Marsden treats patients to medias-
         tinum and supraclavicular regions as well.
      3. Therapeutic questions for discussion.
         a) Can patients with large masses (greater than
            5cm) be treated with abdominal radiation only
            with chemotherapy salvage or possible
            radiotherapy salvage? Should supraclavicular
            and mediastinal XRT be eliminated in this
            subset of patients?

b)  Will CT scanning improve treatment planning
    for patients with large abdominal masses?

Recent data from M.D. Anderson Hospital suggests that
whole abdomen XRT improved outlook for patients with
large masses.

Should patients with large masses be treated with
chemotherapy alone?


C.  Advanced Seminoma

    1.  Nodes above diaphram or visceral diseases.

    2.  General agreement that vinblastine, platinum and
        bleomycin is treatment of choice.


D.  Effect of elevated hCG level on seminoma

    1.  Approximately 9%

    2.  No apparent effect on survival


E.  Post treatment sequelae

    1.  Second testis tumor

    2.  Hypoplastic marrow?  Leukemia?


SUGGESTED REFERENCES

1.  Castro, J.R. and Gonzales, M.:  Results in treatment of
    pure seminoma of the testis. Am. J. Roentgenol. 111:
    355, 1971.

2.  Doornbos, J.F., Hussey, D.H. and Johnson, D.E.:
    Radiotherapy for pure seminoma of the testis.  Radiology
    116:401, 1975.

3.  Doseretz, D.E., et al.:  Megavoltage irradiation for pure
    testicular seminoma:  Results and patterns of failure.
    Cancer 49:2184, 1981.

4.    Earle, J.D., Bagshaw, M.A. and Kaplan, H.S.:
      Supervoltage radiation therapy of the testicular tumors.
      Am. J. Roentgenol. 117:653, 1973.

5.    Javadpour, N.:  Significance of elevated serum
      alphafetoprotein (AFP) in seminoma.  Cancer 45:2116,
      1980.

6.    Javadpour, N., et al.:  The role of alphafetoprotein and
      human chorionic gonadotropin in seminoma.  J. Urol.
      120:687, 1978.

7.    Johnson, D.E., Gomez, J.J. and Ayala, A.G.:  Anaplastic
      seminoma.  J. Urol. 114:80, 1975.

8.    Kademian, M.T., Bosch, A. and Caldwell, W.L.:  Seminoma:
      Results of treatment with megavoltage irradiation.  Int.
      J. Radiat. Oncol. 1:1047, 1976.

9.    Kademian, M., et al.:  Anaplastic seminoma.  Cancer
      40:3082, 1977.

10.   Maier, J.G. and Sulak, M.H.:  Radiation therapy in
      malignant testis tumors part I:  Seminoma; Part II:
      Carcinoma.  Cancer 32:1212, 1973.

11.   Maier, J.G., Sulak, M.H. and Mittemeyer, B.T.:  Seminoma
      of the testis:  Analysis of treatment success and
      failure.  Am. J. Roentgenol. 102:596, 1968.

12.   Quivey, J.M., et al.:  Malignant tumors of the testis:
      Analysis of treatment results and sites and causes of
      failure.  Cancer 39:1247, 1977.

13.   Rosai, J., Silber, I. and Khodadoust, K.:  Spermatocytic
      seminoma:  I. Clinicopathologic study of six cases and
      review of the literature.  Cancer 92, 1969.

14.   Smithers, D., Wallace, E.N.K., and Wallace, D.K.:
      Radiotherapy for patients with tumors of the testicle.
      Br. J. Urol. 43:83, 1971.

15.   Thomas, G., et al.:  Seminoma of the testis:  Results of
      treatment and pattern of failure after radiation
      therapy.  Int. J. Radiat. Oncol. 8:165, 1982.

16. Van der Werf—Messing, B.: Spread of testicular tumours. Clin. Radiol. 22:125, 1971.

17. Van der Werf—Messing, B.: Radiotherapeutic treatment of testicular tumors. Int. J. Radiat. Oncol. 3:235, 1976.

18. Ytredal, D.O. and Bradfield, J.S.: Seminoma of the testicle: Prophylactic mediastinal irradiation versus para aortic and pelvic irradiation alone. Cancer 30:628, 1972.

SECTION V


COMPLICATIONS AND NEW DIAGNOSTIC TECHNIQUES
IN UROLOGIC CANCER


Once cancer has been diagnosed, immediate and intensive treatment is required to ensure greater success in treatment. Unfortunately, intensive treatment (with either surgery, radiation therapy, chemotherapy, or any combination of the three) carries with it another set of problems that, too, may be life-threatening if not controlled properly. This section reviews some common complications resulting from intensive therapy of genitourinary tract cancer. Both antibiotic and cancer chemotherapy-induced nephrotoxicity, radiation therapy complications, and a general chapter on the urologic complications of gynecologic cancers are included and discussed in depth.

Cancer specialists are in agreement that earlier diagnosis of cancer would not only facilitate the subsequent treatment of patients but may also help in controlling and curing cancer. The chapters on therapy-related complications are followed by three chapters looking at new diagnostic techniques in genitourinary cancer. Lymphoscintigraphy may be helpful in assessing pelvic lymph node status in malignancies originating in the genitourinary tract. A new marker for detecting transitional cell carcinoma of the bladder and in vitro clonogenic sensitivity for urologic specimens are discussed in the last two chapters in this section.

CHAPTER 22

ASSESSMENT OF RENAL FUNCTION I - ANTIBIOTIC NEPHROTOXITY IN
THE PATIENT WITH UROLOGIC CANCER


Richard E. Rieselbach



I. MEASUREMENT OF RENAL FUNCTION

The normal kidney carries out complex excretory,
metabolic and endocrine functions that are essential for
homeostasis and are susceptible to impairment in the patient
with urologic cancer. Excretory function is measured by
clinically available laboratory tests which assess glomerular
function, either via direct measurement of glomerular filtration rate (GFR) or by their relationship to GFR. These tests
are useful in clinical management because GFR reflects the
population of functioning nephrons and thus indicates any
functional deficit incurred through loss of nephrons. When
the patient with urological cancer undergoes a loss of nephrons, remaining nephrons become more vulnerable to drug toxicity and pharmacokinetics of many potentially nephrotoxic
drugs, including antibiotics and cancer chemotherapy agents,
are altered. Thus, the dosage of many drugs must be adjusted
according to the degree of functional deficit.

A.  Measurement of GFR

GFR may be estimated by obtaining a timed collection of
urine to determine volume per minute, with analysis of plasma
and urine carried out to determine the concentration of whatever glomerular marker is employed. In practice, a 24-hour
urine specimen is utilized; alternatively, the average of two
2-hour urine collections may be more accurate. An optimal
timed collection of the glomerular marker is achieved by
inducing a water diuresis so as to maximally dilute the marker
and thus minimize any collection error. This may be

163

accomplished by administering a water load of 10 ml/kg approximately one hour prior to the onset of collection, with further administration of water at appropriate intervals. It should be noted that when the serum creatinine is higher than 3 mg/dl, caution must be exercised in administering a water load in order to prevent a dilutional state.

For determination of endogenous creatinine clearance, the patient is instructed to void, and the time of voiding is recorded. Subsequently, all urine voided over the specified time is collected for measurement of volume. At the midpoint of the collection period a plasma sample is collected. The urine and plasma samples are analyzed for creatinine concentration and the clearance is calculated by the formula:

$$\begin{array}{l}\text{Creatinine} \\ \text{Clearance} \\ \text{(ml/min)}\end{array} = \frac{\text{Urine Creatinine}}{\text{Serum Creatinine}} \text{ (mg/dl)} \times \frac{\text{Urine Volume}}{\text{(mg/dl)}} \text{ (ml/min)}$$

The creatinine clearance may be standardized by expressing the clearance in $ml/min/1.73M^2$. The body surface area is estimated from a nomogram of height and weight.

B.  Normal Values for GFR

GFR, as measured by inulin clearance, is remarkably constant in a given individual. Because variation among individuals is substantial, normal values have a wide range. Measurements in normally hydrated young adults adjusted to a standardized body surface area of $1.73M^2$ indicate a mean value for men of 130 ml/min (with a SD of $\pm$ 18%) and 120 ml/min for women (with a SD of $\pm$ 14%). Physiologic variations in GFR occur under a variety of circumstances, such as alterations in blood volume, exercise, and pregnancy.

GFR undergoes a predictable change with age. In the adult, the GFR remains constant until the fourth decade and then gradually declines with increasing age. The kidneys undergo substantial growth from birth to maturity, increasing from an initial two-kidney weight of 50 grams to 270 grams during the third and fourth decades, with a subsequent gradual decline to 185 grams in the ninth decade. The loss of renal mass is mainly cortical and is associated with specific intrarenal vascular changes. This decreasing function with age represents true renal aging and is not secondary to diseases which become increasingly prevalent with progressing age.

This age-related decrease in creatinine clearance is associated with a parallel reduction in daily urinary creatinine excretion. This reflects a decrease in muscle mass and, therefore, a decrease in accession of creatinine to extracellular fluid. A serum creatinine of 1.2 mg/dl may be associated with a GFR of 120 ml/min at age 30, but only 60 ml/min at age 75. Thus, with advancing age, the GFR often undergoes a major decrease, but without an associated increase in serum creatinine. The pharmacologic implications of this decrease in GFR with age are important to the cancer patient because of the many nephrotoxic drugs administered in this setting.

## C.  GFR Within the Single Kidney

The patient who has undergone unilateral nephrectomy sustains only a modest decrease in total GFR, in that the remaining kidney undergoes a substantial increase in GFR per nephron, even in older patients. The major post nephrectomy increase in GFR occurs within three weeks, with GFR increasing to a mean of 66% of the original two-kidney value before nephrectomy. This initial increment occurs regardless of age. In younger patients, a secondary increase occurs over a period of many months. Thus, after unilateral nephrectomy, an older patient might undergo an increase in GFR from 40 to 55 ml/min in the remaining kidney (69% of original two-kidney GFR) as opposed to an increase in a younger patient of 60 to 95 ml/min (79% of original two-kidney GFR). On the basis of the foregoing, if an older patient with kidneys of equal size, who had a GFR of 80 ml/min prior to unilateral nephrectomy, presented 6 months after nephrectomy with a GFR of 40 ml/min, it could be assumed that a significant loss of nephrons had occurred in the remaining kidney due to a pathological process occurring subsequent to nephrectomy. In addition to functional hypertrophy, an actual increase in kidney size occurs following contralateral nephrectomy. This has been demonstrated radiographically and is not related to age. The degree of increase in GFR does not correlate with the increase in kidney size.

## D.  Creatinine Clearance

The endogenous creatinine clearance is the most common method used for measurement of GFR in routine clinical practice. Several aspects of creatinine metabolism allow this solute to be a useful marker of GFR. Creatinine is produced continuously in muscle cells; the rates of production and entry of creatinine into plasma are relatively constant. Thus, in a given individual there is little day-to-day variation in urinary creatinine excretion. For these reasons the concentration of plasma creatinine is relatively constant, allowing utilization of a single plasma sample during a timed collection of urine for the measurement of creatinine clearance.

In health, endogenous creatinine clearance exceeds the simultaneously measured inulin clearance by 5 to 10%. This is because a small amount of creatinine is secreted by proximal tubular cells. A widely used method for measuring creatinine is the Folin picrate ("total chromogen") method, which measures both creatinine and other noncreatinine chromogens. The noncreatinine chromogens account for 5 to 20% of total creatinine concentration at normal levels of plasma creatinine. Since noncreatinine chromogens are not detected in urine, the creatinine clearance estimated by this method is lower than the true creatinine clearance and, fortuitously, is equal to or slightly less than the inulin clearance.

E.  Serum Creatinine

Measurement of serum creatinine concentration is the most commonly used screening test for evaluation of renal function. Under steady-state conditions, the serum creatinine concentration is a function of the rate of creatinine production and excretion. The production of creatinine varies minimally from day to day in any given individual. Thus, since creatinine is excreted primarily by glomerular filtration, the serum creatinine concentration reflects the level of GFR.

In health, serum creatinine concentration as measured by the autoanalyzer technique (total chromogen method) gives a value of $1.1 \pm 0.1$ mg/dl (SD) in males and $0.8 \pm 0.1$ mg (SD) in females. Serum creatinine concentration varies with total muscle mass. Asthenic or cachectic individuals may have values as low as 0.4 to 0.6 mg/dl, whereas in muscular individuals, serum creatinine values as high as 1.4 to 1.6 mg/dl may reflect normal GFR. However, in a given individual the relationship between serum creatinine and GFR is constant and predictable. Having established this relationship, the clinician can estimate serial changes in GFR from measurement of the serum creatinine concentration. Thus, if the serum creatinine concentration is 2.0 mg/dl at a GFR of 60 ml/min,

an increase in serum creatinine concentration from 2 to 4
mg/dl would be expected to represent a reduction of the GFR
from 60 to 30 ml/min. However, this relationship obtains only
if steady-state conditions have been reestablished following
an acute reduction in GFR; otherwise, serious errors may
result from utilizing the serum creatinine as an index of GFR
(i.e., in determining antibiotic dosage). Approximately two
days are required after a 50% reduction in GFR for the serum
creatinine to reach a new steady-state level, thus reflecting
the new level of GFR.

In view of the relationship between serum creatinine and
creatinine clearance depicted in Figure 22-1, it may be
appreciated that nephrotoxicity from a drug may be more
apparent at a higher serum creatinine level. As noted in
Figure 22-1 and Table 22-1, a patient with a serum creatinine

TABLE 22-1

DETECTION OF NEPHROTOXICITY AT TWO
LEVELS OF RENAL FUNCTION

| | BASELINE | | PEAK TOXICITY | | DECREASE |
| | SCr | GFR | SCr | GFR | IN GFR (%) |
| | ml/dl | ml/min | ml/dl | ml/min | |
|---|---|---|---|---|---|
| PATIENT 1 | 1.0 | 100 | 1.5 | 67 | 33 |
| PATIENT 2 | 4.0 | 25 | 6.0 | 17 | 33 |

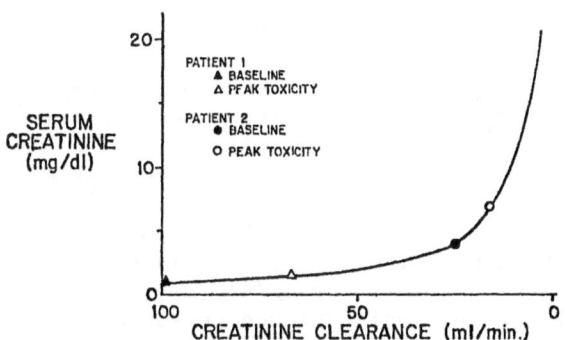

Figure 22-1.  Relationship of serum creatinine to creatinine
clearance (Ref. 10).

of 1.0 mg/dl (representing a GFR of 100 ml/min) may undergo a
33% decrease in GFR and yet sustain an absolute increase in
serum creatinine concentration of only 0.5 mg/dl. By
contrast, a patient with a serum creatinine of 4.0 mg/dl
sustaining the same percentage decrement in GFR would undergo
a 2.0 mg/dl absolute increase in serum creatinine concentration.

F.  Estimation of Creatinine Clearance From Serum
    Creatinine Concentration

When the serum creatinine concentration represents a
steady-state condition, a single serum creatinine value may be
utilized to estimate creatinine clearance. This may be
accomplished by utilizing the following formula developed by
Cockcroft and Gault:

$$\text{Creatinine clearance (ml/min)} = \frac{(140 - age)\,(wt\ in\ kg)}{72 \times serum\ creatinine\ (mg/dl)}$$

The clearance value obtained by this method should be
multiplied by 0.85 in order to correctly estimate GFR in
females. It should be noted that this formula considers body
weight as a variable. The value obtained for creatinine
clearance may be used for calculation of drug dosage, and
should be corrected for body surface area if that is called
for in the particular nomogram utilized to calculate drug
dosage.

G.  Blood Urea Nitrogen

The blood urea nitrogen (BUN) concentration provides a
less reliable estimate of GFR than serum creatinine, in that
urea clearance varies with urine flow and the blood urea
nitrogen concentration is dependent upon nitrogen metabolism
as well as renal function. If these factors are set aside,
the BUN concentration bears a similar relationship to GFR as
serum creatinine. The normal value of BUN varies between 10
and 20 mg/dl in a subject who is well hydrated and ingesting a
normal diet. In this setting, a 50% reduction in GFR would
double the BUN concentration. It should be emphasized that a
normal value of BUN (10 to 20 mg/dl) may reflect a substantial
reduction of GFR in a malnourished person or in a patient with
liver disease. Moreover, the BUN concentration may be
elevated in presence of a normal GFR, if there is coexisting
gastrointestinal bleeding or if corticosteroids or tetra-

cyclines are administered.


## II.   ANTIBIOTIC NEPHROTOXICITY

Infection is a major cause of death in patients with urologic cancer. Attempts to treat these infections lead to the use of a wide assortment of antimicrobial agents, many of which are potentially nephrotoxic. Because cancer patients are often critically ill, broad spectrum coverage with multiple antibiotics is frequently instituted. This, along with the fact that these patients often receive repeated courses of these potential nephrotoxins and are particularly vulnerable to renal damage due to concomitant problems, adds significantly to the risk of severe renal injury in this setting.

Antibiotic nephrotoxicity, with its associated decrease in renal function, greatly complicates the management of the cancer patient, as noted in Table 22-2. Thus, antibiotic nephrotoxicity must be avoided if at all possible; often this may be accomplished by keeping in mind some important preventive considerations as outlined in Table 22-3. In this discussion, we will examine these considerations in more detail, particularly in relation to specific drugs. However, first it is appropriate to consider some general considerations relating to the various types of antibiotic nephrotoxicity which are most commonly encountered.


TABLE 22-2

IMPACT OF RENAL FAILURE ON THE CANCER PATIENT

1.   Alters pharmacokinetics of some anti-cancer drugs.

2.   Superimposes complications of uremia on those of cancer.
     a.   Hemorrhage
     b.   Infection
     c.   Metabolic

3.   Compounds nutritional problems

4.   Additional problems associated with peritoneal or hemodialysis

TABLE 22-3

CONSIDERATIONS IN AVOIDANCE OF NEPHROTOXICITY

1. Awareness of predisposing conditions
   a. Volume depletion
   b. Drug-drug interactions
   c. Pre-existing renal disease
   d. Age

2. Appropriate selection of drugs via knowledge of nephrotoxic potential

3. Appropriate dosing regimens

4. Awareness of early indications of nephrotoxicity and natural history of ARF in this setting

A. General Considerations

The kidney is the primary route of excretion for most of the antibiotics with nephrotoxic potential; during excretion tubular cells are commonly exposed to drug concentrations many times higher than other cells in the body. Conversely, antibiotics which have the liver as their primary mode of metabolism and/or excretion (i.e., clindamycin, lincomycin, erythromycin) are rarely the cause of renal damage. The two major renal pathways for antibiotic excretion are glomerular filtration and tubular secretion. The route of excretion is dependent upon protein binding. An agent such as penicillin, which is 90% bound, is secreted by the proximal tubular organic acid transport mechanism, undergoing minimal filtration. By contrast, aminoglycosides are not protein bound and are excreted exclusively via glomerular filtration. Tubular reabsorption of aminoglycosides normally occurs to only a minor extent; however, this process plays a major role in nephrotoxicity, particularly in those settings where reabsorption is enhanced.

Next, let us consider in some detail those antibiotics which cause acute renal failure. These agents are listed in Table 22-4. Since the aminoglycoside antibiotics, as listed in Table 22-5, represent the most commonly used nephrotoxic antibiotics, nephrotoxicity due to these agents will be considered in some detail.

TABLE 22-4

ANTIBIOTICS CAUSING ACUTE RENAL FAILURE

Aminoglycosides
Cephalosporins
Penicillins
Vancomycin
Trimethoprim-sulfamethoxazole
Pentamidine
Amphotericin-B
Polymyxins
Rifampin
Tetracyclines

TABLE 22-5

AMINOGLYCOSIDE ANTIBIOTICS

1.     Neomycin
2.     Kanamycin
3.     Gentamicin
4.     Tobramycin
5.     Amikacin
6.     Sisomicin
7.     Netilmicin
8.     Streptomycin

B.  Aminoglycosides

     In bacteria, the aminoglycosides penetrate the cell wall
and cytoplasmic membrane; they act on the bacterial ribosomes
causing misreading of the genetic code.  The resulting
synthesis of faulty proteins leads to the death of the micro-
organism.  The polycationic nature of the molecules is responsible for their poor oral absorption, poor penetration into
the cerebral spinal fluid and rapid renal excretion.

     The reported incidence of nephrotoxicity with these drugs
is rapidly rising.  In 1969, the reported incidence of
gentamicin nephrotoxicity was 2 to 3%; in 1979 an incidence
ranging from 16 to 25% was reported.  The reasons for this are
multiple; they include more rigorous criteria for detecting
toxicity, an increase in the recommended dosage, expanding
indications for the use of these drugs, a more resistant

spectrum of gram-negative organisms and frequent utilization
of longer courses of therapy. The clinical hallmark of
aminoglycoside nephrotoxicity is non-oliguric acute renal
failure. In this type of renal failure, the onset is usually
slower and the daily increment of serum creatinine tends to be
less dramatic. Recovery is usually a slow process and may
require more than a month. In some patients, particularly
those with renal impairment prior to receiving the drug,
recovery to baseline function may never occur. Administration
of aminoglycosides may cause enzymuria, proteinuria, amino-
aciduria and glycosuria as a reflection of tubular toxicity.
In actuality, it is likely that all patients receiving
therapeutic doses of aminoglycosides undergo some degree of
nephrotoxicity, as indicated by abnormal excretion of small
molecular weight proteins. Detection of urinary beta-2
microglobulin excretion as well as a urinary concentrating
defect may be the earliest signs of developing nephrotoxicity. It should be recognized that an impairment in glomerular
filtration rate may not be noted until after completion of a
10 to 14 day course of therapy. Some of the risk factors
which enhance the likelihood of developing aminoglycoside
nephrotoxicity are outlined in Table 22-6.

TABLE 22-6

RISK FACTORS FOR AMINOGLYCOSIDE NEPHROTOXICITY

1.  Combination with other nephrotoxins
    a.  Amphotericin
    b.  Cis-platinum
    c.  Radio-contrast media
    d.  Furosemide
    e.  Cephalosporins

2.  Volume depletion - increased tubular reabsorption

3.  Pre-existing renal disease

4.  Age - misinterpretation of serum creatinine

    Since aminoglycoside nephrotoxicity is a dose-duration
phenomenon that occurs in any patient if the exposure is great
enough, proper dosing is essential. Despite the fact that
these agents have been available for over fifteen years, there
is still confusion regarding proper dosing and the use and

meaning of aminoglycoside peak and trough blood levels.
Figure 22-2 represents the excretion curves of netilmicin in
serum following a single 2 mg/kg intramuscular injection in
patients with normal and three levels of reduced renal
function. Note that despite the wide variation in levels of
renal function, peak serum levels consistently fall into the 5
to 7 micrograms/ml range and thus are determined by factors
other than the level of renal function. However, the trough
level is determined by the GFR and the dosing interval chosen
by the physician. Note that for individuals with a GFR of
100, if a dosing interval of every 8 hours is chosen, then the
trough level would be slightly less than 1 microgram/ml prior
to each dose. For individuals with a GFR between 30 and 80
ml/min, approximately 16 hours would be required before the
trough level was below 1 microgram/ml. As can be appreciated,
when the GFR decreases, this curve shifts to the right. Thus,
the biological half-life of aminoglycosides, as with other
drugs excreted by the kidney, is determined by GFR.

Figure 22-3 indicates the two most common approaches
whereby drug dose may be adjusted so as to accommodate for the
impact of GFR upon biological half-life. In this example,
first a dose of 80 mg every 8 hours is depicted in an
individual with a GFR of 100 ml/min. Prior to the dose given
at 8 hours and 16 hours, the trough level is less than 1
microgram/ml. The middle panel shows the excretion curve for

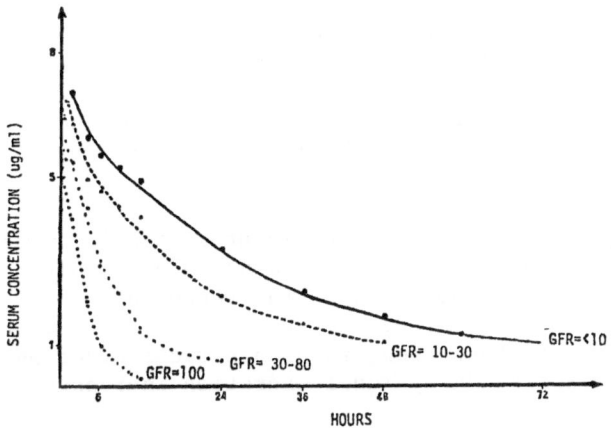

Figure 22-2.   Serum concentration following 2mg/Kg netilmicin
(Ref. 10).

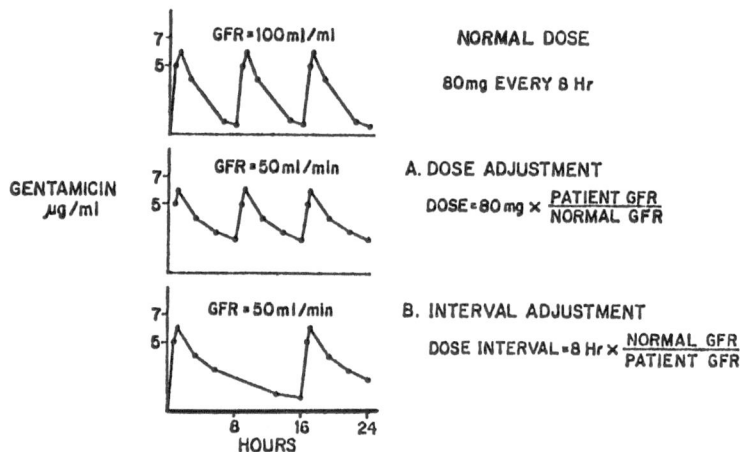

Figure 22-3.   Gentamicin dosing in renal failure (Ref. 10).


gentamicin given to an individual with a GFR of 50 ml/min.
Here the dose reduction approach is utilized, with 40 mg of
drug administered every 8 hours.  Note that peak blood levels
are similar to the patient with normal renal function, but
trough levels are higher as a result of reduced GFR.  The
bottom panel shows the interval adjustment method, where the
dose of drug remains constant but the interval is increased
according to the level of GFR.  This method allows the blood
level to fall to lower trough levels prior to the next dose.
As noted, serum concentration of 5 to 7 micrograms/ml is
reached twice rather than three times during the 24 hour
period.  There are little data favoring one method over the
other.  Most centers employ the interval method because of
greater simplicity of care.

In Figure 22-4, a nomograph is presented for modifying
drug dose or dosage interval according to creatinine clearance
as we have just outlined.  Each line represents one or more
agents, as indicated in the accompanying legend.  Groups of
drugs progress further along in alphabetical order as their
percentage elimination by renal excretion increases.

In utilizing the aminoglycosides, the following guidelines should be applied for safe dosing: 1) The initial dose
should be based on ideal body weight, in an attempt to achieve
the usually recommended therapeutic levels for this particular
drug (i.e.: 5 to 7 micrograms/ml for gentamicin).

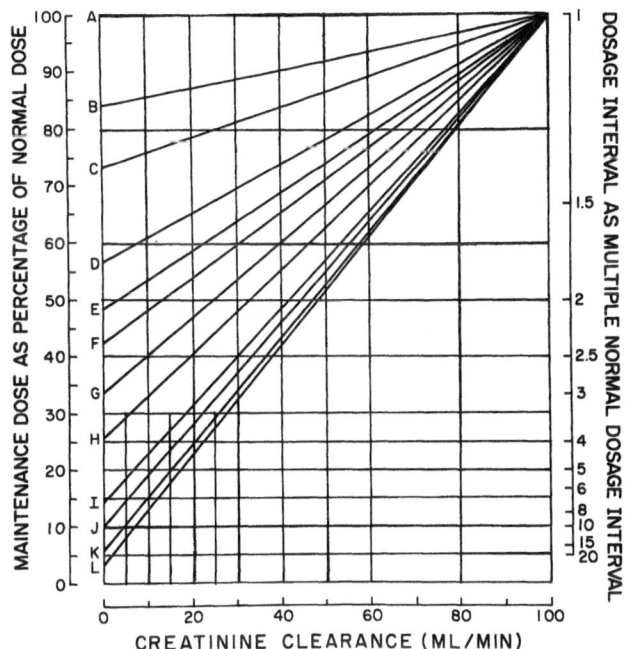

Figure 22-4. Nomograph for modifying drug dose or dosage interval according to creatinine clearance. Each line represents one or more agents:

A  =  minocycline, rifampin
B  =  doxycycline
C  =  clindamycin, chloramphenicol, erythromycin
D  =  isoniazid
E  =  dicloxacillin, sulfadiazine,
       trimethorpim–sulfamethoxazole
F  =  nafcillin, lincomycin
G  =  cefaclor, oxacillin
H  =  cloxacillin
I  =  amoxicillin, cefamandole, methicillin,
       tetracycline
J  =  ampicillin, carbenicillin, cefadroxil,
       colistimethate, penicillin G, ticarcillin
K  =  cefazolin, cefoxitin, cephaloridine, cephalothin,
       gentamicin
L  =  amikacin, cephalexin, flucytosine, kanamycin,
       tobramycin, vancomycin

In patients who have large amounts of adipose tissue, the
actual weight of the patient should not be used to determine
the dosage because aminoglycosides are primarily water soluble
and are distributed in extracellular fluid. 2) Subsequent
dosage should be based upon dose or interval adjustments
according to formulas or nomographs as previously discussed.
It should be emphasized that these methods are merely starting
points and should be followed with peak and trough blood
levels. Peak blood levels should be drawn one hour after I.M.
injection or 15 minutes after I.V. injection. An actual
creatinine clearance is greatly superior to a serum creatinine
level when using the formula or nomographs, particularly if
the serum creatinine level is not stable. 3) Nephrotoxicity is
best detected by observing renal function; trough levels of
aminoglycoside concentration are of less value, in that they
are an indirect indication of renal function. 4) Don't
hesitate to switch to a less nephrotoxic antibiotic if
indicated by subsequent sensitivity results. Remember that
aminoglycosides will ultimately produce nephrotoxicity to some
degree in all patients and should be avoided if less nephrotoxic antibiotics are appropriate.

In the remainder of this presentation, we will briefly
discuss some of the other antibiotics with nephrotoxic
potential.

C. Other Nephrotoxic Antibiotics

1. Polymyxins. When given in doses that result in
blood concentrations of equal antibacterial
effectiveness, the toxicity of colistin and
polymyxin-B are probably similar. In one series,
adverse renal reactions occurred in 20% of patients
receiving these agents. As with aminoglycoside
toxicity, renal function may continue to deteriorate
for a week or more following cessation of therapy
before improvement occurs. Combination of these
agents with cephalosporins appears to enhance the
risk of nephrotoxicity while combination with
aminoglycosides does not. Treatment with these drugs
appears to carry substantially greater risk for
nephrotoxicity than comparable doses of aminoglycosides.

2. Cephalosporins. With the exception of
cephaloradine, these agents have a low potential for

causing nephrotoxicity. Most reported cases of
nephrotoxicity with cephalosporins (other than
cephaloradine) occur when they are used in conjunction with aminoglycosides. However, as previously
discussed, this does not necessarily mean that these
agents themselves are nephrotoxic.

3. <u>Vancomycin</u>. This is a very effective drug when
used against penicillinase-producing staphylococci.
Initially, it was associated with a high incidence of
thrombophlebitis, fever, chills, rash and occasionally nephrotoxicity. Improvements in manufacturing
techniques have eliminated many of these problems, in
that the new preparations are more chemically pure.
Nephrotoxicity from the use of this agent may be a
possibility, but the frequency of its occurrence
appears to be low and certainly considerably less
than that seen with aminoglycoside antibiotics.
However, it should be used cautiously in patients
with reduced renal function, since ototoxicity does
occur with elevated blood levels. Since this drug is
<u>not</u> removed by dialysis it is used frequently in
anephric patients. These patients may be treated
very effectively by giving just one gram per week (15
mg/kg); therapeutic levels may persist for as long as
2 weeks.

4. <u>Trimethoprim-sulfamethoxazole.</u> This drug is
increasingly being used by oncologists in the
prophylaxis and treatment of Pneumocystis carinii
pneumonia. Of course, it is also a very effective
agent in the treatment of urinary tract infections.
This preparation can produce pseudonephrotoxicity, in
that the trimethoprim moiety appears to inhibit the
renal secretion of creatinine, thereby leading to an
elevated serum creatinine concentration in the
absence of a decrease in glomerular filtration rate.
Additionally, one series has described a deterioration of renal function in sixteen patients receiving
TMP-sulfa. Virtually all of these patients had some
underlying renal insufficiency. The sulfa component
of the combination has been thought to be the toxic
element and it is felt that an immunologic or
allergic basis underlies the toxicity. While
crystallization leading to obstructive nephropathy
was a commonly reported complication with early

sulfanilamides, the risk with sulfamethoxazole is minimal.

5. Pentamidine. The use of Pentamidine carries a high risk of renal toxicity, with 24% developing impaired renal function in one series. Since TMP-sulfa is equally effective in treatment of pneumocystis peneumonia, pentamindine should be relegated to a second line status.

6. Amphotericin-B. This antibiotic is used primarily for the treatment of fungal disease and is a well-known nephrotoxin. Toxicity may occur as a result of either intense renal vasoconstriction or binding to tubular cell membranes, resulting in increased cellular permeability and metabolic impairment, particularly of distal tubular cells. The toxic effects of the drug are dose-related, and persistent nephrotoxicity is rare in patients treated with total doses of less than 4 grams. The concomitant use of 5-fluorocytosine has reduced the incidence of nephrotoxicity in patients treated with amphotericin-B by allowing lower doses of amphotericin to be utilized. Patients treated with 0.25 mg/kg/day or less usually tolerate the drug well.

7. Rifampin. While primarily noted for its hepatotoxicity, this drug may also damage the kidneys via the production of acute tubulointerstitial nephritis.

8. Tetracyclines. These drugs are well known to increase BUN as a result of their anti-anabolic action; they do not produce direct renal toxicity. However, the exacerbation of an already present azotemic state may lead to an increase in uremic gastrointestinal symptoms, causing ECF volume depletion and thus a further decrease in renal function. An increase in BUN has not been observed with doxycycline, one of the newer tetracycline analogues. Thus, this drug is the tetracycline of choice for patients with underlying renal impairment.

D. Acute Tubulointerstitial Nephritis (ATIN)

This entity, the second most commonly encountered antibiotic-induced renal disorder, is characterized by

peristent fever, eosinophilia and skin rash, as well as other
features (Table 22-7).  A similar picture may be induced by
ampicillin, naficillin, oxicillin, carbenicillin, and some

TABLE 22-7

Summary of Pertinent Clinical and Laboratory Data in 14
Patients with Methicillin-induced Interstitial Nephritis+

| DATA | % OF PATIENTS |
|---|---|
| Methicillin therapy | |
| Average dose methicillin (g/day) | 8.07 |
| Average total dose methicilin (g) | 124 |
| Average day of methicillin therapy when reaction detected | 12 |
| | |
| Earliest detected manifestation | |
| Fever | 58 |
| Hematuria and pyuria | 14 |
| Elevated serum creatinine | 14 |
| Eosinophilia | 7 |
| Rash | 7 |
| | |
| Clinical finding during course of syndrome | |
| Fever | 100 |
| Rash | 29 |
| Arthralgia | 7 |
| Oliguria | 29 |
| Anuria | 21 |
| | |
| Laboratory findings during course of syndrome | |
| Increased peripheral eosinophil count | 100 |
| Eosinophiluria | 100* |
| Pyuria | 100 |
| Hematuria | 93 |
| Proteinuria | 36 |
| Bacteriuria | 0 |
| Elevated serum creatinine level | 100 |

*Nine of nine patients studied
+Linton, A.L., et al: Acute interstitial nephritis due to
drugs. Ann. Intern. Med., 93:735, 1980.

of the cephalosporins and sulfonamides. One particular
clinical feature that helps identify this disorder is
defervescence from the fever of the primary disease followed
by a second febrile episode due to the drug reaction. Also,
in contrast to aminoglycoside nephrotoxicity, severe renal
dysfunction often requiring hemodialysis treatment is not
uncommon. It should be emphasized that eosinophiluria (i.e.:
eosinophiles comprising greater than 33% of urinary white
cells) is a very helpful laboratory finding. When an air-
dried urinary sediment is stained with Wright's stain,
eosinophiles in the urine appear as granulated, binucleated
cells, which, even if they do not take up the eosine stain,
may be distinguished from polymorphonuclear leukocytes or
lymphocytes by their bilobed appearance. This form of
toxicity, which appears to have a delayed type of hypersensi-
tivity as its basis, will frequently respond to discontinuing
the drug. However, if full-blown oliguric acute renal failure
occurs, it would appear that recovery may be substantially
accelerated by prednisone therapy.

E.  Glomerular and Vascular Reactions

Very rarely, penicillins have been implicated in the
development of acute glomerulonephritis, often associated with
a generalized vasculitis. In these cases, the dose of
penicillin has been low and occasionally toxicity has followed
a single dose. Also, a disorder resembling periararteritis
nodosa has been reported following exposure to sulfathiazole.

SELECTED REFERENCES

1.  Mazumdar, D.C. and Rieselbach, R.E.: Diagnostic approach
    to renal disease. In: Rieselbach, R. and Garnick, M.B.,
    eds, Cancer and the Kidney. Philadelphia: Lea and Febiger,
    1982, p.3.

2.  Row, J.W. et al.: The effect of age on creatinine
    clearance in man: A cross-sectional and longitudinal
    study. J. Gerontol. 31:155, 1976.

3.  Boner, G. et al.: Factors influencing the increase in
    glomerular filtration rate in the remaining kidney of
    transplant donors. Am. J. Med. 55:169, 1973.

4.  Boner, G., Sherry, J. and Rieselbach, R.E.: Hypertrophy of
    the normal human kidney following contralateral
    nephrectomy. Nephron 9:364, 1972.

5.  Kassirer, J.P.: Clinical evaluation of kidney function.
    Glomerular function. N. Engl. J. Med. 285:385, 1971.

6.  Brodey, M. and Craig, W.: Antimicrobial-induced renal
    failure; choice of antimicrobials in renal insufficiency
    and/or urinary tract infection. In: Rieselbach, R.E.  and
    Garnick, M.B., eds. Cancer and The Kidney. Philadelphia:
    Lea and Febiger, 1982, p. 824.

7.  Appel, G.B. and Neu, H.C.: The nephrotoxicity of
    antimicrobial agents. New Engl. J. Med., 296:663, 1977;
    296:722, 1977; 296:784, 1977.

8.  Porter, G.A. and Bennet, W.M.: Toxic Nephropathies. In:
    Brenner, B. and Rector, F., eds. The Kidney. Philadelphia,
    W.B. Saunders Co., 1981, p. 2045.

9.  Cronin, R.E.: Antimicrobial agent nephrotoxicity. In:
    Anderson, R. and Schrier, R. eds. Clinical Use of Drugs in
    Patients with Kidney and Liver Disease.  Philadelphia:
    W.B. Saunders Co., 1981, p. 54.

10. Cronin, R.E. Antibiotic-induced renal diseases.
    University of Texas Southwestern Medical School, Medical
    Grand Rounds, October 9, 1980.

CHAPTER 23

ASSESSMENT OF RENAL FUNCTION II - CANCER CHEMOTHERAPY INDUCED
NEPHROTOXICITY

Marc B. Garnick

The kidney is extremely susceptible to toxic damage from a
variety of sources. The commonly-used antineoplastic agents
can induce renal injury by themselves, as well as causing
additive or synergistic toxicity when used in addition to
radiation therapy. Likewise, the concomitant presence of
hypercalcemia, hyperuricemia, or urinary tract obstruction may
enhance the renal damage from a variety of therapeutic modalities. This section will highlight the frequently
encountered renal complications of cancer therapy as it
relates to chemotherapy. The clinician must be constantly
aware of newly introduced cancer chemotherapeutic agents, as
the list of renally toxic compounds will undoubtedly grow as
more agents are introduced into clinical trials.

CIS-PLATINUM

Cis-diamminedichloroplatinum(II) has recently been introduced with an antineoplastic spectrum of activity in the
treatment of genitourinary cancer. The compound has become a
major component of combination chemotherapy programs in
treating metastatic gonadal germ cell cancer, ovarian cancer,
bladder carcinoma, squamous cell carcinoma of the head and
neck, non-oat cell lung cancer, as well as other gynecologic
neoplasms. In addition to nephrotoxicity, a variety of
non-renal side effects occur and include hematologic and
gastrointestinal toxicity, ototoxicity, anaphylaxis, nephrotoxicity in the form of peripheral neurophathy, hyperuricemia,
and occasionally seizures and other miscellaneous phenomena.

183

Preclinical Studies

Drug-induced renal damage remains one of the most critical
side effects of cis-platinum in preclinical small and large
animal toxicology studies. Pathologically, the morphologic
alteration resulting from cis-platinum included epithelial
cell degeneration and proximal tubular necrosis. While
proteinuria commonly occurs, glomerular damage was unusual in
these preclinical studies. Physiologically, cis-platinum in
animal studies has induced an uncoupling of renal mitochondrial oxidative phosphorylation and disrupted proximal tubular
cell energy production shortly after drug administration.
Additional abnormalities include defects in medullary solute
acccumulation leading to concentrating abnormalities, as well
as the development of renal insensitivity to vasopressin in
the collecting tubule.

Pharmacology

In pharmacologic studies, intravenous bolus administration
of platinum has revealed a $T_{1/2}$ alpha ranging between 25-49
minutes, with a $T_{1/2}$ beta between 58-73 hours. Ninety percent of the drug is protein bound to albumin, gamma globulin
and transferrin. Urinary excretion accounts for 27-50% of the
drug, usually within 5 days following administration. There
is a prolongation of the $T_{1/2}$ beta in patients with renal
insufficiency. Tissue distribution studies have shown that
following cis-platinum administration, highest tissue levels
are seen immediately in the plasma and kidney, followed by the
gonadal tissue. Levels in the renal medulla and renal cortex
persisted for greater than 6-7 days in both animal and human
studies.

Clinical Studies of Nephrotoxicity

Human investigations of cis-platinum nephrotoxicity have
demonstrated histopathologic changes consisting of renal
cortical swelling, medullary congestion, and focal coagulative
necrosis of the distal convoluted tubules and collecting
ducts. Tubular dilitation of the convoluted segments in the
distal tubule, atypical epithelial cells with syncitial nuclei
and granular casts have also been noted. These changes,
however, are not specific for cis-platinum nephrotoxicity. In
physiologic evaluations of renal function in patients

TABLE 23-1. Cis-Platinum Nephrotoxicity in Early Phase I Studies (Reproduced with permission, Lea and Febiger, Philadelphia, Ref. 3.)

| Cis-platinum dose and schedule (mg/M²) | N (pts) | % Developing nephrotoxicity ⊕ | Comments |
|---|---|---|---|
| 50 IVB⊕ or 10 dx5⊘ | 25 | 24 | peritoneal dialysis required in several patients |
| 75 IVB or 15 dx5 | 14 | 14 | hyperuricemia noted in 16/60 courses |
| 100 IVB or 20 dx5 | 18 | 61 | renal bx in 2 pts: acute tubular necrosis tubular degeneration interstitial edema |
| 200 IVB | 1 | 100 | |
| 50 IVB q̄ 2 wks | 3 | 100 | |
| 75 IVB q̄ 2 wks | 3 | 67 | |
| 100 IVB q̄ 2 wks | 9 | 100 | 5/9 pts at 100 mg/M² dose had irreversible nephrotoxicity |
| 18 IVB dx5 q̄ 3 wks | 5 | 20 | led to ATN⊘ in 2 pts |
| 20 IVB dx5 q̄ 3 wks | 9 | 33 | |
| 24 IVB dx5 q̄ 3 wks | 3 | 100 | |
| 15 IVB dx5 q̄ month | 10 | 30 | renal toxicity thought to be cumulative |
| 17.5 IVB dx5 q̄ month | 5 | 60 | nephrotoxicity greatest 3 weeks after drug administered |
| 15 twice weekly | 13 | 31 | |
| 30 dx3⊘ q̄ 4 wk ("high dose") | 13 | 54 | 1-2 liters NSS⊕ after each dose ovarian cancer patients significant nephrotoxicity in "high dose" group |
| 30 d 1, q̄ 2-3 wk ("low dose") | 19 | 5 | "low dose" devoid of significant nephrotoxicity 1-2 liters NSS after treatment |

⊕ IVB - intravenous bolus
⊘ dx5 - daily dose for 5 consecutive days
⊘ dx3 - daily dose for 3 consecutive days

⊕ % developing nephrotoxicity refers to % of patients. In many instances, the percentage cited aplies to % of courses as well
⊘ ATN - acute tubular necrosis
⊕ NSS - normal saline solution

receiving cis-platinum, serial determinations of serum creatinine and glomerular filtration rate (GFR) demonstrated
transient falls in the GFR, but usually with full recovery by
day 21.  It should be mentioned that these studies occurred
after saline hydration had been instituted.

When cis-platinum was initially introduced as a phase I
agent (Table 23-1), nephrotoxicity seemed to be the dose
limiting toxicity.  Indeed, the incidence of renal damage in
patients receiving a variety of cis-platinum dosages and
schedules ranged from between 50-100% of patients treated.  In
renal biopsy specimens obtained from several patients, acute
tubular necrosis, tubular degeneration, interstitial edema,
and fatal acute renal failure ensued.  From the early studies,
it was concluded that renal toxicity was probably cumulative,
and nephrotoxicity seemed to be most profound 3 weeks after
the drug was administered.  It must be emphasized, however,
that little, if any attention was paid to the hydration status
of the patients receiving the drug.  Indeed, many patients
experienced profound nausea and vomiting secondary to
cis-platinum, became dehydrated, and had inadequate access to
fluid.  This combination of factors almost undoubtedly
accounted for the high incidence of renal damage in early
studies.

Later phase I and phase II studies emphasized the importance of saline hydration, with or without diuretic agents
(Table 23-2).  Thus, the majority of later investigations
using cis-platinum were accompanied by a marked dimunition in
the number of patients and percent of courses associated with
cis-platinum nephrotoxicity.  A variety of hydration schedules
have been used, including 3-6 liters of normal saline per day,
with or without mannitol or furosemide diuretic administration.  All factors such as extracellular fluid volume expan-
sion with saline hydration, accompanying diuretic administration, and rate of drug administration have contributed to a
lowered incidence of nephrotoxicity.  Still, the optimal drug
schedule and method of administration remain to be defined.
The schedules appear equal in their ability to prevent
nephrotoxocity, provided that the hydration status is closely
monitored and adequate urinary output is maintained.  While
some investigators suggest the addition of mannitol or loop
diuretics to the hydration schedule, others feel that the
clinical utility of these agents in further preventing
nephrotoxicity is not proven.  Obviously, clinical trials will
have to assess the importance of both osmotic and loop

diuretics within optimal hydration regimens.

Protection from cis-Platinum Nephrotoxicity: Experimental Data

From an experimental viewpoint, a variety of pharmaco-
logical interventions have been used to modulate the nephrotoxocity of cis-platinum. Agents such as Probenecid, the
radioprotective agent, WR2721, diethyldithiocarbamate, and
sodium thiosulfate have all been used in preclinical animal
studies and have shown some efficacy in further diminishing
the renal damage secondary to cis-platinum administration.

METHOTREXATE

Methotrexate, one of the most commonly used chemotherapeutic agents, is ordinarily excreted by the kidneys. In the
face of compromised renal function, serum levels of methotrexate remain elevated and bone marrow depression, mucositis,
and dermatitis ensue. While nephrotoxicity is rare after
conventional dosing in patients with previously normal renal
function, one series of 13 patients with advanced cancer
resulted in elevation of the BUN in 5 patients. Two of these
5 patients died with persistent azotemia and 1 patient demonstrated direct renal tubular damage at the time of post mortem
examination. This was characterized by extensive necrosis of
the convoluted tubular epithelium.

In the past, far higher doses of methotrexate (1-7.5
$gm/M^2$ i.v., weekly) have been used in the management of
patients with various cancers. Although controversy surrounds
the permanent role of high dose methotrexate (followed by
citrovorum factor rescue) in the management of patients with
neoplastic diseases, it is commonly being used at several
institutions for a variety of indications. When methotrexate
is given in high doses, nephrotoxicity has been a prominent
side effect which, on occasion, has limited its usefulness.
Although the exact pathogenesis of methotrexate-induced renal
failure has not been fully delineated, several mechanisms have
been proposed. These include precipitation of the antifol in
the renal tubules, a direct toxic effect of methotrexate on
renal tubules, and direct effects of methotrexate on the
glomerular filtration rate.

In earlier clinical studies which evaluated high dose

TABLE 23-2. Cis-platinum Nephrotoxicity: Influence of infusion duration and Hydration/Diuretic Regimens (Reproduced with permission, Lea and Febiger, Philadelphia, Ref.3)

| Cis-Platinum Dosage and Schedule (mg/M²)[1] | Hydration | Diuretics | No. of Patients | Nephrotoxicity % Patients | Nephrotoxicity % Courses | Comments |
|---|---|---|---|---|---|---|
| 5 over 30 min, then 20 Cl[2] d × 5[3] q 3-4 weeks | 3-6 l[5]/day | — | 33 | 21 | 11 | decreased gastrointestinal (GI) toxicity nephrotoxicity not progressive |
| 50-130 over 24 hr | 6 L/day then 150 ml/hr for 24 hr | — | 18 | — | 6 | decreased GI toxicity most patients received 80 mg/M² |
| 3-5 mg/kg IVB[6] over 10-15 min ("high dose") (120 IVB) | • 2 l D5 ½ NSS[8] 12 hr pre-plat • then 200 ml D5 NSS/hr × 6 hr • then input = output | • 12.5 g mannitol' pre-plat • then 10 g/hr × 6 hr | 52 | 19 | — | 9/10 patients who developed Cr[9] ≥ 2 mg/dl had preexisting renal dysfunction with CrCl[10] of 50-70 ml/min |
| 20-40 Cl daily for 5 d | • 1 L D5 ½ NSS pre-plat • p.o. intake to insure 2 L fluid/d | • furosemide 40 mg daily × 5d | 30 | 17 | 13 | marked decrease in GI toxicity nephrotoxicity developed in 5 patients: 4 treated at 35-40 mg/M²/d × 5d (cumulative dose 175-200 mg/M²); 1 treated at 20 mg/M²/d × 5d (cumulative dose 100 mg/M²) |
| 20 over 2 hr, d × 5 | • 125 ml/hr NSS × 12 hr pre-plat • then 125 ml/hr NSS × 5 days | — | 25 | 15 | — | all elevations in Cr reversible no patient had increase in Cr ≥ 25% above baseline testis cancer patients |

| Dose | Hydration | Diuretic | | | Comments |
|---|---|---|---|---|---|
| 20 over 15 min, d×5 | • 100 ml/hr NSS × 12 hr pre-plat  • then continuous saline hydration at 100 ml/hr of NSS × 5 days | — | 47 | "rare" | no patients developed Cr ≥ 1.5 mg/dl testis cancer patients |
| 70 over 30–60 min | • IV hydration④ pre-plat × 12 hr  • 200 ml/hr D5 ½ NSS × 5 hr after plat  • then additional IV hydration for 12 hr | • 40 mg furosemide and 37.5 g mannitol 1 hr pre-plat  • 50 g mannitol after plat over 5 hr | 25 | 34 | — | ovarian cancer patients |
| 20 over 1–2 h, d×5 | 1 L NSS pre-plat | — | 15 | — | 47 | GFR⑧ measured with ¹²⁵iothalamate; transient diminution in 47% courses, with subsequent full recovery patients with marginal CrCl (17–45 ml/min/M²) did not experience a deterioration in renal function after receiving additional cis-platinum |
| 1 mg/kg over 6 hr twice weekly then q̄ 3 weeks  60 over 6 hr twice weekly then q̄ 3 weeks | • 1 L D5 NSS pre-plat  • 2 l D5 1/3 NSS during cis-platinum, given over 6 hr  • then intake = output | • 37.5 g mannitol  • 40 mg furosemide | 18 | 21 | — | 21% patients developed transient, reversible drops in CrCl |
| | | | 6 | ↑ | | all renal parameters returned to baseline within 28 d |

①All dosages in mg/M² unless otherwise indicated (all dosages of cis-platinum are in boldface type)
②Cl—continuous infusion
③d×5—daily dose for 5 consecutive days
④IVB—intravenous bolus
⑤L—liters
⑥D—dextrose
⑦NSS—normal saline solution; cis-platinum should be diluted in a solution with a high ambient chloride concentration, e.g. normal saline solution or D5 ½ NSS, but not D5 W.
⑧Nonspecified
⑨Cr—serum creatinine
⑩CrCl—creatinine clearance
⑪GFR—glomerular filtration rate
Plat—cis-platinum
q̄—every

TABLE 23-3

High Dose MTX Nephrotoxocity - Early Studies

| Creatinine Increase (%) | Patients (N=33) | | Courses (N=72) | |
|---|---|---|---|---|
| | N | % | N | % |
| 25-50 | 5 | 13 | 13 | 18 |
| >50 | 19 | 60 | 21 | 29 |
| | 24 | 73 | 34 | 47 |

methotrexate, the hydration status and extracellular fluid
volume status of patients were not well assessed. Results of
such studies are seen in Table 23-3.

In early studies, a 50% elevation from the baseline serum
creatinine has been reported in 60% of patients 24 hours after
receiving high doses of the drug. Three of 33 patients
included in the early studies died with acute renal failure.
Post mortem examination of kidneys demonstrated bilateral
renal enlargement, methotrexate precipitation in the tubules,
and native methotrexate within the renal parenchymal tissue.
In recent studies, in which vigorous urinary alkalinization
and hydration programs have been employed, the incidence of
nephrotoxicity in 178 patients fell markedly. Thirty patients
(17%) developed creatinine increases of greater than 50% but
less than 100% above baseline, and only 6 patients (3%)
developed increases in their creatinine of greater than 100%
above baseline. In the extensive experience using high dose
methotrexate with "rescue" at the Sidney Farber Cancer
Institute, 1216 courses have been evaluated and moderate or
severe nephrotoxicity occurred in only 7% of such courses, as
seen in Table 23-4. Doses of MTX ranged between 1 and 7.5
$gm/M^2$ i.v. weekly.

The overall treatment plan for patients who do develop
methotrexate-induced renal toxicity includes the following:

1) In anticipation of giving high dose methotrexate, the
patient should be vigorously hydrated with between 3-5
liters of $D_5W$ containing 60 mEq/liter of sodium
bicarbonate. Hydration generally begins 12-14 hours
prior to initiating methotrexate and should continue

TABLE 23-4

High Dose MTX Nephrotoxicity - Recent Studies

| Creatinine Increase (%) | Patients (N=178) N | % | Courses (N=1216) N | % |
|---|---|---|---|---|
| >50   ≤100 | 30 | 17 | 85 | 7 |
|        | 6 | 3 | 6 | <1 |
| >100 | 36 | 20 | 91 | 7 |

for at least 2-3 days following the end of the methotrexate infusion.

2) A basal GFR and serum creatinine should be obtained prior to administering methotrexate.

3) Prior to initiating therapy, the urinary pH should be maintained at about 7. Therapy should be withheld until this urine pH has been obtained. Twenty four hours after the completion of methotrexate administration, a repeat serum creatinine should be obtained and compared to the post-hydration, pre-treatment baseline level.

4) If the serum creatinine rises by 50% or more from the baseline level, this usually indicates renal toxicity. If this occurs, citrovorum factor should be continued at usual doses in these patients until the methotrexate level falls below $7.5 \times 10^{-8}$M. Hydration and alkalinization should be maintained during this period of evaluation.

5) If the serum creatinine rises 100% or more at the 24 hour point, acute renal failure usually ensues. The urinary alkalinization and hydration should be maintained as before. In addition, citrovorum factor dosages should be increased from 15 mg to 150 mg every 3 hours. Consideration should be given to the addition of thymidine as well.

These supportive measures are continued until the serum methotrexate level is less than $10^{-7}$M, and the serum creatinine has normalized, which can take up to 30-60 days. A full discussion of all of the biochemical rescue techniques is beyond the scope of this section. The reader is referred to reference 3 for a detailed discussion.


NITROSOUREAS


Streptozotocin (Streptozocin) (Table 23-5)

The nitrosourea streptozotocin has recently been approved by the FDA for marketing in the United States for a variety of indications. The drug has a role in the management of patients with metastatic islet cell carcinoma of the pancreas, carcinoid, and several other cancers. Preclinical studies of animal toxicity included nephrotoxicity as the prominent side effect. A variety of non-specific pathologic changes have been noted, including vacuolization and PAS positivity in the proximal tubular cells, and mitochondrial disruption. In addition, several animal investigations have also indicated that streptozotocin may indeed be an inducer of renal tumors in several species.

A variety of renal and metabolic abnormalities have been reported following the administration of streptozotocin in man. Nephrotoxicity is the principle side effect which limits the usefulness of this drug. Fanconi syndrome, hypophosphatemia, glycosuria, proteinuria, renal tubular acidosis, low serum bicarbonate, hypokalemia, and nephrogenic diabetes insipidus have all resulted with a reasonable degree of frequency. Hypophosphatemia and proteinuria are the usual first manifestations of renal toxicity and require meticulous attention to renal status before additional drug is administered. Most worrisome, however, is the development of azotemia, increase in serum creatinine and dimunition of serum creatinine clearance, which have occurred in approximately 20-40% of patients treated over a prolonged period. Indeed, life threatening and fatal renal failure has occurred in approximately 5% of patients reported in the literature. In this group of patients, acute tubular necrosis was demonstrated at the time of autopsy. Although a variety of schedules have been employed, one recommendation calls for 1.5 $gm/M^2$/week or 0.5 $gm/M^2$ days 1-5 repeated every 3-4 weeks. Streptozotocin is not recommended in patients with pre-existing renal dysfunction.

TABLE 23-5. Streptozotocin Nephrotoxicity (Reproduced with permission, Lea and Febiger, Philadelphia, Ref. 3)

| Toxic Effect | Dosage and Schedule | | | Overall N (%) | Comments |
|---|---|---|---|---|---|
| | A: 0.6-2 g/M²/wk[1] N (%) | B: 1.5-7.5 g/M²/wk or 0.1-1.6 g/d × 5 q̄ 2 wk N (%) | C: 0.5g/M²/d × 5 q̄ 6 wk N (%) | | |
| Fanconi syndrome | 24/64[2] (38) | — | — | 24/64 (38) | Hypouricemia, aminoaciduria have both been reported |
| Hypophosphatemia | 33/69 (48) | 7/54 (13) | — | 40/123 (33) | Hypophosphatemia may be first abnormality (with proteinuria) and usually occurs after 1-2 drug courses |
| Glycosuria | 27/69 (39) | 11/107 (10) | — | 38/176 (22) | Usually not related to hyperglycemia |
| Proteinuria | 57/101 (56) | 34/107 (32) | — | 91/208 (44) | Proteinuria usually first manifestation of renal toxicity; best monitor for development of more significant renal toxicity; withhold drug until proteinuria reverses. |
| Renal tubular acidosis | 18/64 (28) | 8/99 (8) | — | 26/163 (16) | Lactic acidosis 2° to STZ due to decrease in lactate metabolism, has also been reported[11] |
| Low serum bicarbonate | 6/51 (12) | 11/65 (17) | — | 17/116 (15) | |
| Hypokalemia | 16/69 (23) | — | — | 16/69 (23) | Hypocalcemia has also been reported |
| Nephrogenic diabetes insipidus | — (1-2) | — (1-2) | 1/74 (1-2) | — (2) | |
| Azotemia[3] ↓ CrCl[4]; ↑ Cr[5] | 35/96 (36) | 27/132 (20) | 21/74 (28) | 83/302 (27) | |
| Life-threatening/fatal renal failure | 9/131 (7) | 4/106 (4) | 1/74 (1) | 14/311 (5) | Acute tubular necrosis demonstrated from autopsies of patients Recommended STZ doses: 1.5 g/M²/wk or 0.5 g/M² d × 5 q̄ 3-4 wk STZ not recommended in patients with preexisting renal dysfunction |

[1] majority of patients in this schedule received 1-1.5 g/M² weekly, for 4-6 weeks
[2] number developing toxic effect/number evaluated
[3] majority of cases with BUN > 25 mg/dl; 30-50% fall in CrCl; serum Cr > 1.8 mg/dl
[4] CrCl—creatinine clearance
[5] Cr—serum creatinine

Methyl-CCNU
(1-(2-chloroethyl)-3-(4-methylcyclohexyl)-1-nitrosourea)

Methyl-CCNU has recently been identified as a potential
nephrotoxin, both in pediatric and adult patients treated for
a variety of neoplasms. In several recent reports, the
development of chronic renal failure was observed in 6
children who received greater than 1500 mg/$M^2$ of methyl-CCNU
generally given over a period of 17 months. In a review from
the Mayo Clinic, an incidence of 2.1% of nephrotoxocity was
observed in 857 consecutive adult patients treated with
methyl-CCNU either as a single agent, or in combination
chemotherapy programs.

The clinical syndrome surrounding renal damage from
methyl-CCNU is associated with a diminution in renal size as
the major manifestation. Pathologically, the most prominent
renal changes consist of glomerular sclerosis with thickening
of the glomerular basal membrane and severe nephron loss.
Other changes include interstitial fibrosis and cellular
infiltration. While pathologically the lesion of nitrosourea
nephrotoxicity may resemble radiation nephropathy, the
clinical syndromes are really quite different.

While formal recommendations can not be made with
certainty regarding the use of nitrosoureas, it seems prudent
to limit the use of methyl-CCNU to doses less than 1200
mg/$M^2$ and treatment courses of less than 1 year. Obviously,
patients undergoing such therapy should have serial renal
ultrasound examinations and periodic determinations of renal
function. Therapy should be terminated at the first sign of
diminution in renal size.

Mitomycin-C

Recent studies have noted a questionable association of
mitomycin-C therapy with subsequent nephrotoxicity. However,
patients on chronic therapy with mitomycin-C, especially those
combination programs which contain a nitrosourea, should be
followed closely for the development of nephrotoxicity.

Other renal-related toxicities of mitomycin-C include a
symptom complex consistent with the hemolytic-uremic syndrome.

MISCELLANEOUS AGENTS

A variety of other antieoplastic agents have been associated with nephrotoxicity. These include mithramycin, during its use as an anticancer agent in patients with germ cell carcinoma of the testis. Renal function should be monitored carefully in patients receiving lower doses of mithramycin for the management of malignant hypercalcemia, as abnormalities in renal function may occur even with these lower dosages. 5-Azacytidine has been associated with renal tubular dysfunction and a spectrum of proximal and distal tubular abnormalities. However, a clear cut relationship between drug and the development of nephrotoxicity is not well established. Other agents such as doxorubicin (Adriamycin) and cancer immunotherapy with C-parvum have been associated with a spectrum of renal abnormalities in case report forms.

SUGGESTED REFERENCES

1. Rieselbach, R.E. and Garnick, M.B., eds.: Cancer and the Kidney. Philadelphia: Lea and Febiger, 1982.

2. Garnick, M.B. and Mayer, R.J.: Management of acute failure associated with neoplastic disease. In: Yarbro, J. and Bornstein, R., eds. Oncologic Emergencies. New York, Grune & Stratton, Inc. p. 247, 1981.

3. Abelson, H.T. and Garnick, M.B.: Cancer chemotherapy induced acute renal failure. In: Rieselbach, R.E. and Garnick, M.B., eds. Cancer and the kidney. Philadelphia, Lea & Febiger, 1982, p. 769.

4. Frei, E. III, et al.: High dose methotrexate with leucovorin rescue: Rationale and spectrum of antitumor activity. Am. J Med. 68:370, 1980.

5. Rozencweig, M., et al.: Cis-diamminedichloroplatinum(II), a new anticancer drug. Ann. Intern. Med. 86:803, 1977.

6. Anderson, T. et al. Proceedings of the National Cancer Institute conference on cis-platinum and testicular cancer. Cancer Treat Rep. 63:1431, 1979.

7.  Prestayko, A.W., Crook, S.T. and Carter, S.K., eds:
    Cisplatin - Current status and new developments. New York
    Academic Press, 1980.

8.  Blachley, J.D. and Hill, J.B.: Renal and electrolyte
    disturbances associated with cisplatin.  Ann Intern Med.
    95:628, 1981.

9.  Weiss, R.B.: Streptozocin: A review of its pharmacology,
    efficacy, and toxicity. Cancer Treat.Rep. 66:427, 1982.

10. Harmon, W.E. et al.: Chronic renal failure in children
    treated with methyl-CCNU. N.Engl.J.Med. 300:1200, 1979.

CHAPTER 24

UROLOGIC COMPLICATIONS OF GYNECOLOGIC CANCERS

Gary P. Kearney

I. GYNECOLOGIC ANATOMY

A. Structural Relationships

1. Cervix and bladder separated only by a layer of
   pubovesical fascia
2. Ureter passes less than 1 cm from cervix
3. Ureter may be closely associated with the ovary
   if there are adhesions between the ovary and
   peritoneum

B. Blood Supply

1. Bladder--superior and inferior vesical arteries
2. Ureter (in female)--internal iliac, uterine, and
   inferior vesical arteries
3. Ovaries--ovarian artery
4. Fallopian tubes--uterine and ovarian arteries
5. Uterus--uterine and ovarian arteries
6. Vagina--vaginal artery and branches of the
   uterine, middle rectal, and internal pudendal
   arteries

C. Lymphatic Drainage

1. Ovary--para-aortic nodes
2. Uterine fundus (segments) and Fallopian
   tubes--para-aortic or pelvic nodes
3. Cervix and lower uterus--parametrial, internal
   iliac, and obturator nodes and then to the

197

external iliac nodes; cervix also drains to the
presacral nodes
4. Vagina--upper part, external and internal iliac
nodes; lower part, superficial inguinal nodes


II.  UROLOGIC INVOLVEMENT IN GYNECOLOGIC CANCER

A. Cancer of the Cervix

1. Responsible for 6% of cancer in women and 5% of
female cancer mortality
2. Gynecologic neoplasm that most frequently
involves the urinary tract
3. Death most often results from uremia secondary to
ureteral obstruction
4. Mechanisms of ureteral obstruction
a.  Direct extension--first to adventitia, then
muscularis,and finally mucosa
b.  Compression by tumor-filled lymphatics--
usually where ureter passes through the
cardinal ligament, 3 to 6 cm from the
ureterovesical junction

B. Cancer of the Uterus
1. Carcinoma

a.  Responsible for 13% of cancer in women
b.  Lower incidence of urinary tract involvement
than cancer of the cervix
i.   Bladder involvement rare
ii.  Ureteral and urethral obstruction
somewhat more common
2. Sarcoma
a.  Responsible for about 1% of cancer in women
b.  Highly invasive; spreads hematogenously
c.  Mesenchymal sarcoma, in its more
differentiated form, may involve the urinary
tract

C. Cancer of the Ovary

1. Fourth leading cause of death among cancers in
women
2. Ureteral compression frequent
a.  Via displacement of bladder anteriorly

      b. From extension to pelvic and para-aortic
        lymph nodes


III. DIAGNOSTIC ASSESSMENT OF THE URINARY TRACT

  A. Purpose

    1. To determine whether the urinary tract is
       involved in the cancer
    2. To assess renal function
    3. To define any congenital urinary tract anomalies
       before surgery
    4. To assess symptoms of ureteral obstruction after
       treatment

  B. Excretory Urography

    1. Most important technique in these patients
       because of the morphologic and functional
       information given
    2. Follow-up studies allow an assessment of the
       significance of any urinary tract abnormalities

  C. Isotope Renography

    1. Sensitive and specific indicator of obstruction
    2. Cannot provide morphologic detail
    3. Used mostly for serial follow-up

  D. Computed Tomography

    1. Can image ureteral involvement
    2. Differentiation of recurrent tumor and radiation
       fibrosis may be difficult

  E. Ultrasonography

    1. Useful for evaluating tumor extension and for
       detecting hydronephrosis
    2. Particularly suited for serial evaluations

  F. Diagnostic Thin-Needle Biopsy of Ureteral
    Obstruction

    1. May avoid needless surgery in patients with

recurrent disease

G. Cystoscopy

   1. Necessary in all patients with cervical cancer
      a. In stage I and II disease to rule out
         associated bladder pathology
      b. In stage III and IV disease for precise
         staging
   2. Useful after radiation therapy if urinary
      symptoms have developed
   3. Best performed under general or regional
      anesthesia in patients with known tumor
      involvement of the bladder

H. Retrograde Pyelography

   1. Can provide detailed information on ureteral
      obstruction that may not be obtainable by
      excretory urography
   2. Should be approached with extreme caution
      a. Contrast injection beyond a high-grade
         obstruction can lead to sepsis and
         pyonephrosis
      b. Placement of a ureteral catheter for
         decompression may then be necessary or
         surgical intervention if that is not
         successful

IV. URINARY TRACT INVOLVEMENT IN EXTENSIVE OR RECURRENT
    DISEASE

   A. Ureteral Obstruction

      1. Most common urinary tract complication of
         gynecologic cancers
      2. Usually involves distal ureter
      3. Obstruction of proximal ureter alone is possible
         if tumor has metastasized to lymphatics outside
         the pelvis before there is extensive intrapelvic
         involvement
      4. Clinical findings
         a. Classic symptom: dull, constant ache in lower
            lumbar region or groin that may be referred
            to the flank, lower abdomen, thigh, or leg

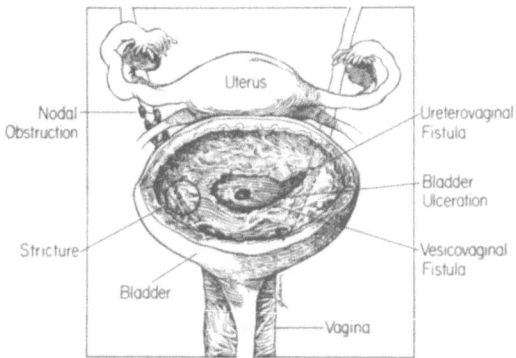

Figure 24-1. Involvement of the urinary tract by gynecologic cancers. The bladder may be subject to direct extension of the tumor, ulceration following radiation therapy, or vesico-vaginal fistula following radiation therapy or surgery. The ureters may be invaded by tumor or compressed by the tumor-filled lymph nodes. Ureteral stricture or uretero-vaginal fistula formation may follow radiation therapy or surgery. In the diagram, the anterior wall of the bladder is cut away to show several of these possible complications. (Reproduced with permission, Lea and Febiger, Philadelphia, Ref. 11).

        b.  Irritative symptoms possible if there is an associated infection
        c.  Almost half of patients may be asymptomatic
        d.  Found at diagnosis in about 15% of patients
        e.  Incidence correlated with increasing stage of disease
     5. Prognosis
        a.  When found at diagnosis, is a poor prognostic sign
        b.  Following treatment, usually indicates recurrent tumor, which is often unresectable

B. Bladder Invasion

     1. Occurs less frequently and at a later clinical stage than does ureteral obstruction

2. Most common in carcinoma of the cervix
3. Extension of cervical carcinoma to the bladder in
   the absence of distant metastases does not
   preclude a good outcome


V.  UROLOGIC COMPLICATIONS OF RADIATION THERAPY

A. Incidence

   1. Has been decreasing over time, reflecting
      modifications in technique
   2. Is less than 5% for major complications
   3. Is far less than the incidence of urinary
      complications due to recurrent disease

B. Factors Predisposing to Complications

   1. Most injuries are caused by treatment errors or
      repeated irradiation for persistent or recurrent
      disease
   2. Tissue health may be a factor
      a. Hypertension and diabetes have been found to
         be associated with fistula development after
         irradiation
   3. Urinary tract infections are a risk factor

C. Types of Complications

   1. Ureteral Obstruction
   2. Bladder ulceration
      a. Ulcers are usually single, in the
         supratrigonal area, and from millimeters to 4
         cm, in size
      b. Biopsy may be required, but occasionally even
         histologic examination may not be able to
         distinguish radiation necrosis from tumor
   3. Fistulas
      a. May be either ureterovaginal or vesicovaginal
      b. Predisposing factors
         i.  High-dose radiation
         ii. Ureteral or bladder invasion by tumor,
             since tumor necrosis after irradiation
             can result in a tissue deficit
   4. Kidney damage
      a. A small reduction in glomerular filtration

rate may result

VI.  UROLOGIC COMPLICATIONS OF SURGICAL TREATMENT

A. Types of Operations

   1. Total abdominal extrafascial hysterectomy
      a.  Performed for in situ and stage IA carcinoma
          of the cervix
      b.  Involves removal of the cervix and adjacent
          tissues as well as the upper vagina in a
          plane outside the pubocervial fascia
      c.  Causes minimal disturbance of the ureters and
          trigone of the bladder
   2. Modified radical hysterectomy
      a.  Also performed for microinvasive carcinoma of
          the cervix
      b.  Includes, in addition, dissection of the
          ureters in the paracervical tunnel with
          removal of parametrium and paracervical
          tissue medial to the ureter
   3. Radical abdominal hysterectomy with bilateral
      pelvic lymphadenectomy
      a.  Performed for stage IB and IIA carcinoma of
          the cervix
      b.  Includes a wider resection of the
          paracervical tissues, involving mobilization
          of the bladder neck and dissection of the
          ureters
      c.  Carries risk of ureterovaginal and
          vesicovaginal fistulas

B. Types of Complications

   1. Bladder injuries
      a.  Direct--usually on posterior bladder wall,
          above and between the ureteral orifices,
          where the vaginal cuff is sutured
      b.  Neurologic--may occur during radical
          hysterectomy
   2. Ureteral injuries
      a.  Intraoperative--usually involve lower third
          of ureter
      b.  Obstruction after operation
          i.  Transient--usually from postoperative

edema, infection, and impaired lymph
flow
ii. Chronic--from devascularization of the
distal ureters or from inadvertent
inclusion in a bulk ligature
3. Fistulas
a. Ureterovaginal, the more common type, occur
after 4 to 10% of radical hysterectomies
b. Predisposing factors
i. Cancers of higher stage
ii. Previous radiation therapy
iii. Postoperative urinary tract infection

VII. MANAGEMENT OF INTRAOPERATIVE COMPLICATIONS

A. Bladder Injuries

1. Recognition
a. Intraoperative recognition is extremely
important
b. Techniques
i. Preoperative placement of a three-way
catheter allowing intraoperative filling
of the bladder with sterile normal
saline colored with indigo carmine or
methylene blue
ii. Cystography before catheter removal
2. Repair
a. In absence of previous radiation therapy--
layered bladder closure without tension,
extraperitoneal drainage, and Foley catheter
and/or suprapubic catheter drainage
b. In patients with previous radiation
therapy--use of omentoplasty as adjunct may
avoid the possibility of a vesicocutaneous
fistula.

B. Ureteral Injuries

1. Recognition
a. Can prevent kidney damage or fistula
formation
b. Occurs intraoperatively in only 30% of cases
2. Repair
a. Limited in situ repairs

       i. Patient must be without history of radiation therapy or ureteral devascularization

      ii. Simple suture ligature repaired by ligation and placement of an inlying ureteral stent

  b. More extensive repairs

       i. Necessary if ureter has been transected

      ii. May require ureteroureterostomy and/or ureteral reimplantation

     iii. If ureteral division is low in pelvis, ureteral reimplantation is safest

     iv. A Boari bladder flap and/or nephropexy may be employed in the reimplantation

VIII. MANAGEMENT OF RADIATION AND DELAYED SURGICAL COMPLICATIONS

A. <u>Ureteral Stricture</u>

  1. Treatment options

    a. Cystoscopic introduction of an internal ureteral stent

    b. Ureteroneocystostomy with ureteral stent, with or without Boari flap

    c. Transureteroureterostomy

    d. Creation of a high urinary conduit

B. <u>Bladder Ulceration</u>

  1. Cystectomy and urinary diversion control hemorrhage but may carry high risk in elderly population

  2. Alternatives may be instillation of 10% formalin, alcohol, or phenol, or hydrostatic intravesical pressure therapy

C. <u>Ureterovaginal Fistulas</u>

  1. Diagnosis

    a. Sign: spontaneous drainage of urine from the vagina, usually with ureteral obstruction

    b. Ureter involved can be determined by excretory urography

  2. Treatment

      a. Resembles that carried out for ureteral
         stricture
      b. In the absence of flank pain, treatment can
         be delayed; multiple attempts at ureteral
         stent placement may be successful
      c. Watchful waiting may allow spontaneous
         closure

D. Vesicovaginal Fistulas

  1. Diagnosis
      a. Sign: spontaneous drainage of urine from the
         vagina
      b. Can be confirmed by dye cystography, using a
         vaginal tampon to demonstrate staining
      c. Excretory urography may show a characteristic
         double-contrast appearance
      d. Cystoscopy can demonstrate size and
         appearance of the fistula
      e. Biopsy of vaginal apex and margins of the
         fistula is necessary to eliminate possibility
         of recurrent tumor
  2. Treatment
      a. In patients without history of radiation,
         repair is made 3 to 6 months after operation
         to avoid possible surgical failure
      b. Spontaneous healing may occur
      c. Suprapubic approach preferred unless fistula
         is low and small
      d. Steps
         i. Separation of the fistula from the
           bladder wall by wide mobilization,
           division of all adhesions, and excision
           of devascularized tissue
        ii. Interposition of additional layers of
           tissue; use of peritoneum, omentum,
           gracilis muscle, or labial fat pad
           important in irradiated patients
        iii. Placement of temporary splinting
           catheters in the ureters can avoid
           kinking and postoperative ureteral edema
           if the fistula is near the ureteral
           tunnel
        iv. Urethral catheter drainage preferred
           during healing

IX. URINARY DIVERSION

   A. Indications

      1. As part of a pelvic exenterative procedure for
         treatment of recurrent or extensive disease
      2. For palliation of symptoms of urinary tract
         complications
         a. In patients with intractable vesicovaginal
            fistulas, severe radiation cystitis, or
            extensive bladder scarring after radiation
            resulting in urinary incontinence

   B. Results

      1. Palliative diversion in patients with
         tumor--patients have a limited lifespan after
         diversion and are denied a painless uremic death

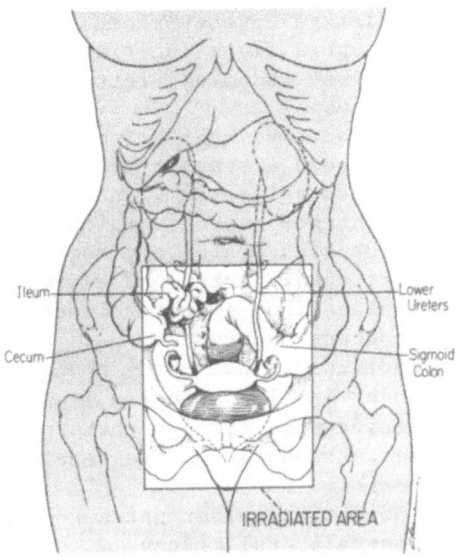

Figure 24-2. The unshaded area indicates the organs subject
to irradiation, the use of which should be avoided in urinary
reconstruction or diversion whenever possible. (Reproduced
with permission, Lea and Febiger, Philadelphia, Ref. 11.)

2. In the absence of persistent tumor, diversion and
   exenteration are successful techniques

C. <u>Techniques</u>

   1. Transureteroureterostomy
      a. Indications: ureteral obstruction and
         impaired functioning of the nonobstructed
         kidney in a patient with an irradiated
         bladder
      b. Contraindications: infection, calculus
         disease, retroperitoneal fibrosis,
         tuberculosis
      c. Frozen sections of the ureter used for the
         anastomosis should be examined to rule out
         cancer
      d. The ureter should cross above the inferior
         mesenteric artery, and the anastomosis should
         be tension-free
   2. Cutaneous ureterostomy
      a. Indications: stable, poor-risk patient with a
         short life expectancy
      b. Unilateral ureterostomy is carried out
         through a flank incision and an upper
         anterior abdominal retroperitoneal stoma is
         created
      c. Nephrectomy, angiographic infarction, or
         cutaneous ureterostomy may be indicated in
         the contralateral kidney
      d. Advantages over diversion through a bowel
         segment: ureterostomy does not involve
         peritoneal cavity and avoids potential
         leakage from a ureterointestinal anastomosis
   3. Percutaneous nephrostomy
      a. Indication: emergency procedure performed
         under local anesthesia
      b. Drainage is through catheter inserted
         percutaneously in the renal pelvis
   4. Nephrectomy
      a. Indication: older patient with a normal
         contralateral kidney
   5. Transverse colon conduit/jejunal conduit
      a. Indications: patients undergoing pelvic
         exenteration as well as selected patients
         treated by urinary diversion alone who have
         previous or planned extensive irradiation

   b. Transverse colon is most often used since it
      lies outside the irradiated field, but either
      ileum, jejunum, or occasionally high sigmoid
      colon may be used
   c. In a patient with a trained sigmoid colostomy
      who requires urinary diversion, a jejunal
      loop should be considered to avoid a wet
      colostomy

SELECTED REFERENCES

1. Lang, E.K., et al.: Complications in the urinary tract
   related to treatment of carcinoma of the cervix. South.
   Med. J. 66:228, 1973.

2. Walsh, J.W., et al.: Recurrent carcinoma of the cervix:
   CT diagnosis. Amer. J. Roentgen. 136:117, 1981.

3. Richie, J.P., Withers, G., and Ehrlich, R.M.: Ureteral
   obstruction secondary to metastatic tumors. Surg.
   Gynecol. Obstet. 148:355, 1979.

4. Van Dyke, A.H. and van Nagell, J.R., Jr.: The prognostic
   significance of ureteral obstruction in patients with
   recurrent carcinoma of the cervix uteri. Surg. Gynecol.
   Obstet. 141:371, 1975.

5. Dean, R.J. and Lytton, B.: Urologic complications of
   pelvic irradiation. J. Urol. 119:64, 1978.

6. Mattingly, R.F. and Borkowf, H.I.: Acute operative injury
   to the lower urinary tract. Clin. Obstet. Gynecol. 5:123,
   1978.

7. Keetel, W.C., et al.: Surgical management of
   urethrovaginal and vesicovaginal fistulas. Am. J. Obstet.
   Gynecol. 131:425, 1978.

8. Mahoney, E.M., Kearney, G.P., and Prather, G.C.: Improved
   non-intubated ureterostomy technique for the normal and
   dilated ureter. J. Urol. 117:279, 1977.

9. Hodges, C.V., et al.: Transureteroureterostomy: 25-year
   experience with 100 patients. J. Urol. 123:834, 1980.

10. Schlesinger, R.E.: et al.:  The choice of an intestinal
    segment for a urinary conduit.  Surg. Gynecol. Obstet.
    148:45, 1979.

11. Kearney G.P. and Knapp, R.C.:  Genitourinary complications
    of Gynecologic Cancers.  In:  Rieselbach, R.E. and
    Garnick, M.B., eds. Cancer and the Kidney, Philadelphia:
    Lea and Febiger, 1982, p. 742.

CHAPTER 25

RADIATION THERAPY COMPLICATIONS OF THE GENITOURINARY TRACT

William D. Bloomer

KIDNEY

Knowledge of radiation damage to the kidney assumes particular importance today as successful treatment programs evolve which combine radiation therapy with potentially nephrotoxic chemotherapy. In addition, tumor infiltration, obstructive uropathy and metabolic derangements associated with the primary cancer itself can compromise renal function before the initiation of radiation treatments.

The response of the normal kidney to irradiation can be classified by histological changes, physiological alterations and clinical sequelae. Although the majority of patients treated with abdominal and retroperitoneal radiation therapy do not clinically manifest overt kidney damage, sequential function and pathologic alterations do occur.

Histologic Changes

Most animal and human data indicate that fractionated doses of 1000-2000 rad over a period of 2-3 weeks to all of both kidneys do not produce any sustained pathologic abnormalities. With doses of 2300-2500 rads over 4-5 weeks, early radiation histopathological changes can be detected and have been termed "nephroglomeruloendotheliosis". The histologic changes are diffuse and initially affect endothelium of the glomerulus and the glomerular afferent arterioles. Endothelial swelling accompanied by hyaline deposition in the intima and medial layers of arterioles leads to glomerular capillary swelling, edema and eventual occlusive changes in the

211

capillary loops. An occasional tubule may become atrophic,
but the major lesions involve afferent arterioles and
glomerular endothelium. Although most of these changes are
reversible at these dose levels, some nephrons will be
permanently damaged and may be forerunners of the patchy
parenchymal lesions seen in late radiation nephritis.

The late histologic manifestations of radiation injury,
many of which are related to the development of hypertension,
closely resemble the changes associated with arteriolar
nephrosclerosis, chronic glomerulonephritis, and pyelonephritis. Late radiation nephrosclerosis constitutes a specific
entity and is characterized by the following criteria:
1. Reduction in renal parenchymal mass secondary to
   nephron atrophy.
2. Capsular thickening and fibrosis associated with a
   "pebbled" renal surface.
3. Vascular changes:
   a. Prominent interlobular and arcuate arteries with
      sclerosis
   b. Hyalinization and occlusion of afferent arterioles
   c. Occlusion of glomerular capillary loops with
      glomerular hyalinization and prominent mesangial
      cells.
   d. Efferent arteriole and interstitial capillary
      necrosis with tubular atrophy and progressive
      interstitial fibrosis.
4. Relative lack of inflammatory cell infiltrate.

## Physiological Studies

Although common renal function tests show no consistent
changes with doses up to 2400 rad to all of both kidneys,
alterations in glomerular filtration rate (GFR), renal plasma
flow (RPF) and tubular excretory capacity have been reported.
GFR was transiently reduced after 400 rad, normal or slightly
elevated after 1625 rad and decreased with higher doses. RPF
fell consistently after 400-750 rad. Tubular function as
measured by para-amino hippurate was not consistently reduced
until higher doses of irradiation were delivered. Despite
reductions in GFR and RPF to values as low as 40 percent of
control values, all patients were clinically normal.

## Clinical Syndromes

Acute radition nephritis is characterized by signs and

symptoms of renal and cardiovascular dysfunction and is
temporally related to the exposure of the kidneys to therapeutic radiation. Acute clinical changes occur between 6-12
months after irradiation and do not become important until at
least 2300-2500 rads have been delivered to the whole of both
kidneys, usually over a 5 week period of time. In its acute
form, pedal edema, dyspnea on exertion, headache, and nocturia
are accompanied by hypertension, cardiac enlargement, anemia,
and proteinuria. The syndrome can progress to a full-blown
hypertensive encephalopathy and chronic renal failure, and
pathophysiologically is related to the hypertension component. Patients who develop malignant hypertension have a poor
prognosis. The etiology of the hypertension may be related
initially to alterations in the juxtaglomerular apparatus and
an increased vascular sensitivity which perpetuates the
hypertension--renal damage cycle. A normochromic normocy-
tic anemia may be present and is also a poor prognostic sign.
While the kidneys may seem to recover and the hypertension
regress, this is not usually the case. Of the 20 patients
with acute radiation nephritis reviewed by Luxton, 6 of 8
patients with malignant hypertension died within 3-12 months,
and 10 of the 20 patients ultimately died. The fatal cases
showed a combination of hypertensive encephalopathy, left
ventricular failure, congestive heart failure and uremia. The
early deaths were due to hypertensive disease and later deaths
to uremia. Full recovery rarely occurs after acute radiation
nephritis, and patients who survive the acute phase are
generally left with decreased renal function progressing to
chronic radiation nephritis.

The chronic form of radiation nephritis usually occurs
after a period of time (6-18 months) during which the patient
remains asymptomatic. Patients may be found to have symptomatic renal failure (usually chronic). The chronic form may
also be insidious, and patients may present with asymptomatic
renal failure. A history of acute renal damage is not a pre-
requisite for chronic radiation nephritis. Estimates of renal
tolerance are derived from the observation of Luxton and
Kunkler after large abdominal field irradiation for patients
with seminoma of the testis. When doses of 2500-3250 rads
were delivered over 3-6 weeks to all of both kidneys, 40%
developed renal damage, and 13% died. Of those patients with
chronic radiation nephritis, the majority developed the
clinical picture of chronic glomerulonephritis. Asymptomatic
proteinuria has been observed over a period of many years
following renal irradiation. It may be intermittent and

mild. Standard renal function tests are often normal, but a
latent type of nephritis may develop with impaired renal re-
serve and occasional elevation of blood urea nitrogen.

Although hypertension may be present, it is not a
necessary accompaniment. Some patients may be normotensive
for years and complain only of lack of energy and nocturia.
In Luxton's series of 24 patients with chronic radiation nephritis, 9 had normal blood pressure for an average of 8 years.
The outlook in those who survived from acute radiation nephritis was better than in patients in whom the development of
nephritis was insidious. Of 14 patients with secondary
chronic radiation nephritis, 9 led normal lives for periods up
to 11 years after radiotherapy. Some patients who are otherwise asymptomatic may develop a benign form of hypertension
accompanied by variable proteinuria developing 6-12 months
after irradiation. Although most patients in this group do
well, a few may progress to malignant hypertension even after
a period of many years. Malignant hypertension can be fatal
in a few weeks as hypertensive encephalopathy and brain stem
hemorrhage develop. There may be associated papilledema, re-
tinitis and a rising blood urea nitrogen. In patients with
known chronic radiation nephritis or benign essential hypertension, the malignant hypertension may develop over a period
of years.

Treatment

     The natural history of radiation nephritis before dialysis
or transplantation came into general clinical practice was one
of progressive renal failure and death. The majority of
patients, however, recovered but with varying degrees of
hypertension and diminished renal function. If hypertension
results from unilateral renal damage, surgical removal of the
affected kidney has occasionally resulted in clinical
improvements.

     The best treatment, however, is prevention, i.e,, adequate
renal localization and limitation of dose and volume. The
threshold for irreparable damage to all of both kidneys is not
clearly defined; however, 2000 rads in 10 fractions over 2
weeks is generally regarded as a very safe treatment plan. It
is not uncommon to exceed this dose to one kidney in the
treatment of upper abdominal malignancies. Provided the dose
to one kidney does not exceed 2000 rads in 10 fractions, dose
to the other kidney is limited by gastrointestinal tolerance.

Further definitions of renal tolerance are conjectural.

## Combined Modality Therapy

The enhancement of radiation damage by actinomycin D has become a well recognized complication of multimodality cancer treatment. In these studies, radiation nephritis occurred at lower kidney radiation doses when chemotherapeutic agents were used concurrently. Although the increased toxicity could not be quantitatively expressed, the oncologist should be well aware of this potential danger with actinomycin D and other drugs.

## URETERAL TOLERANCE

Ureteral injuries secondary to radiation therapy are rare (less than 1%), take the form of strictures generally at the ureterovesical junction, and occur 6 months to several years after treatment. They usually occur as sequelae to treatment for cervix cancer where external beam irradiation has been combined with intracavitary radium application. Sequential intravenous pyelography at yearly intervals for 2-3 years should be routine in patients treated for cervix cancer. The major differential diagnosis is recurrent tumor. The diagnosis must often be established by laparotomy. The simplest treatment is a ureteral stent but reimplantation or diversion may be necessary. Nephrostomy should be reserved for patients with renal pelvic distention, sepsis with hydronephrosis or advancing uremia. Nephrectomy is indicated with recurrent sepsis. Urinary diversion in the face of recurrent tumor should be undertaken only after careful assessment of the patient's disability and life expectancy.

## BLADDER TOLERANCE

Acute radiation cystitis develops after external beam radiation doses of 3000 rads. Dysuria, frequency and nocturia are characteristic symptoms; diffuse hemorrhage is rare. Cystoscopy findings vary with the severity of reaction but early findings are hyperemia and occasional petechiae. These acute symptoms are usually self-limiting and are best treated symptomatically with pyridium or Ditropan, a reduction in daily dose fraction size or a short treatment break.

Chronic radiation cystitis develops 4-12 months after irradiation but longer symptom-free intervals are not

uncommon. Painless hematuria with or without hemorrhage are
classical presentations. The recurrence and severity of these
late complications are not necessarily related to either acute
symptom severity or radiation dosages less than 7000 rad
external beam or 10,000 mg. hr radium exposure. The incidence
of late bladder injuries is less than 5%. Cystoscopy reveals
tuft-like or tortuous blood vessels with erythema, bullous
edema at sites of inflammation or bleeding ulceration. The
epithelium otherwise is usually pale, atrophic and has a fine
telangiectatic pattern. Histologically, interstitial fibrosis
and endarteritis obliterans are the predominant lesions seen.
Hyalinazation of the muscularis with fibrosis and vascular
sclerosis are also common. Bladder contraction is more likely
when surgery has been performed in conjunction with
irradiation.


SUGGESTED REFERENCES

1.  Garnick, M.B. and Mayer, R.J.:  Acute renal failure
    associated with neoplastic disease and its treatment.
    Semin. Oncol. 5:155, 1978.

2.  Richie, J.P. and Garnick, M.B.:  Primary renal and
    ureteral cancer, In:  Rieselbach, R.E. and Garnick, M.B.,
    eds.:  Cancer and the Kidney, Philadelphia: Lea & Febinger,
    p. 662., 1982.

3.  Maier, J.G.:  Effects of radiation in kidney, bladder and
    prostate.  Front. Radiat. Ther. Oncol. 6:196, 1972.

4.  White, D.C.:  The histopathologic basis for functional
    decrements in late radiation injury in diverse organs.
    Cancer 37:1126, 1976.

5.  Kunkler, P.B., Farr, R.F. and Luxton, R.W.: The limit of
    renal tolerance to x-rays: An investigation into renal
    damage occurring following the treatment of the tests by
    abdominal baths. Br. J. Radiol. 25:190, 1952.

6.  Luxton, R.W.: Radiation nephritis, Quart. J. Med. 22:215,
    1953.

7.  Luxton, R.W. and Kunkler, P.B.: Radiation nephritis. Acta
    Radiol (Stockholm) 2:169, 1964.

8.  Rubenstone, A.I. and Fitch, L.B.: Radiation nephritis.  A clinicopathologic study. Am. J. Med. 33:545, 1962.

9.  Levitt, W.M.: Radiation nephritis. Br. J. Urol. 29:381, 1957.

10. Avoili, L.V., et al.: Early effects of radiation on renal function in man. Am. J. Med. 34:329, 1963.

11. Sagerman, R.H.: Radiation nephritis. J. Urol. 91:332, 1964.

12. Cassady, J.R., et al.:  Considerations in the radiation therapy of Wilms' tumor.  Cancer 32:598, 1973.

13. Arneil, G.L., et al.:  Nephritis in two children after irradiation and chemotherapy for nephroblastoma.  Lancet 1:960, 1974.

14. Churchill, D.N., Hong, K. and Gault, M.H.:  Radiation nephritis following combined radiation and chemotherapy (bleomycin-vinblastine).  Cancer 41:2162, 1978.

15. Kottmeier, H.L.:  Complications following radiation therapy in carcinoma of the cervix and their treatment. Am. J. Obstet. Gynecol. 88:854, 1964.

16. Slater, J.M. and Fletcher, G.H.:  Ureteral strictures after radiation therapy for carcinoma of the uterine cervix. Am. J. Roentgenol. 111:269, 1971.

17. Watson, E.M., Herger, C.C. and Sauer, H.R.:  Irradiation reactions in the bladder.  Their occurrence and clinical course following the use of x-ray and radium in the treatment of female pelvic disease. J. Urol. 57:1038, 1947.

18. Strockbine, M.F., Hancock, J.E. and Fletcher, G.H.: Complications in 831 patients with squamous cell carcinoma of the intact uterine cervix treated with 3000 rad or more whole pelvis irradiation. Am. J. Roentgenol. 108:293, 1970.

19. Galleher, E.P., Jr., et al.:  A follow-up study of supervoltage irradiation followed by cystectomy for bladder cancer. J. Urol. 99:59, 1968.

SECTION VI


EPIDEMIOLOGY AND MISCELLEANOUS SITES


The last section concludes with a discussion of two very rare genitourinary tract cancers, cancer of the adrenal cortex and cancer of the penis.  Chemotherapy and surgery both play a role in the treatment of the two, with surgery being the most successful in cancer of the adrenal cortex.  A combination of chemotherapy and surgery with radiotherapy is generally employed in the management of penile cancer.

The epidemiology of urologic cancers is presented, and, finally, a look at new directions in medical oncology, with a specific discussion of new and advanced treatment modalities for genitourinary cancer, concludes the proceedings.

CHAPTER 26

NEW DIAGNOSTIC TECHNIQUES - LYMPHOSCINTIGRAPHY


William D. Kaplan



The non-surgical techniques currently available for assessing pelvic lymph node status in malignancies originating in
the colon and rectum, bladder, prostate, and testes are not
sufficiently accurate as to completely obviate the need for
surgicopathological staging.  A newer radiologic test may
offer a diagnostic alternative.

Radionuclide lymphoscintigraphic results following interstitial radiocolloid injection in the evaluation of the internal mammary lymph nodes suggest a clinically acceptable level
of sensitivity and specificity for detecting tumor involvement
within lymph nodes.  The technique has recently been applied
to the demonstration of pelvic and abdominal lymphatics, channels which are not routinely identified during conventional
bipedal lymphangiography.

Selection of the optimal radiocolloid injection site for
defining pelvic lymphatic drainage was based upon early observations following injection of supravital dye into the lower
third of the rectum.  The dye injection technique allowed
definition of lymphatic channels which approximated the anatomic pathway of ischiorectal fossa lymph drainage terminating
in the external, internal, and common iliac lymph nodes.  It
was assumed, therefore, that by substituting a radiocolloid
for the dye and injecting perianally, one could visualize and
externally image nodal drainage pathways from the ischiorectal
fossa.  This would therefore allow the clinician to assess
potential sites of neoplastic spread in patients with malignancies of the lower rectum and adjacent pelvic organs.

The technique is easily performed. The patients is placed in the lithotomy position, and the perianal region cleansed twice with a Betadine solution. The skin is dried, and approximately 0.2 ml of technetium-99m-antimony sulfide colloid* is deposited into the ischiorectal fossa bilaterally, using a tuberculin syringe fitted with a 22 gauge 1 1/2" needle. For the injection, the syringe is held parallel to the table top, and the needle is inserted to its full length. No local anesthesia is needed since the procedure meets with excellent patient tolerance.

Images are obtained on a standard Anger (gamma) camera, fitted with a low energy all purpose parallel hole collimator. Immediately following the injection, a 500,000 count anterior view of the pelvis is obtained to delineate the configuration of the injectate. Three hours post injection, a similar 500,000 count image of the injection site is obtained, along with 100,000 count anterior, posterior, and lateral images of the pelvis and abdomen.

A normal lymphoscintigraphic scan is defined as visualization of lymph nodes in sequence which evidence a relatively symmetric uptake of radiocolloid. Although there is some variation in the number of nodes visualized and the relative degree of radiocolloid sequestration, this general pattern of bilateral symmetry and uniform uptake has been a reliable indicator of the absence of lymph node involvement by tumor (Fig. 26-1).

Abnormal uptake can be manifested as (a) impeded flow from the injection site, (b) decreased regional uptake of radiocolloid within individual nodes, or (c) involvement of an entire lymphatic chain (Fig. 26-2).

The results of iliopelvic lymphoscintiscans as correlated with the stage of disease in 170 patients with diverse pelvic malignancies are seen in Table 26-1. The trend is predictable in that patients with more extensive primary malignancies and those with recurrent tumor have a greater frequency of either unilaterally or bilaterally abnormal lymphoscintigraphic studies.

* Cadema Medical, Inc., PO Box 97, Westtown, NY  10998

TABLE 26-1

RESULTS (%) OF ILIOPELVIC LYMPHOSCINTIGRAPHY ACCORDING
TO STAGE OF DISEASE IN 170 PATIENTS WITH
DIVERSE PELVIC MALIGNANCIES (10)

|  | Primary | Extensive Primary | Recurrent With & Without Metastases |
|---|---|---|---|
| Bilateral Normal | | | |
| Unilateral S A A ⎱ | 35 | 29 | 28 |
| Bilateral S A A ⎰ | 63 | 64 | 72 |

S = Suspicious
A = Abnormal or Absent

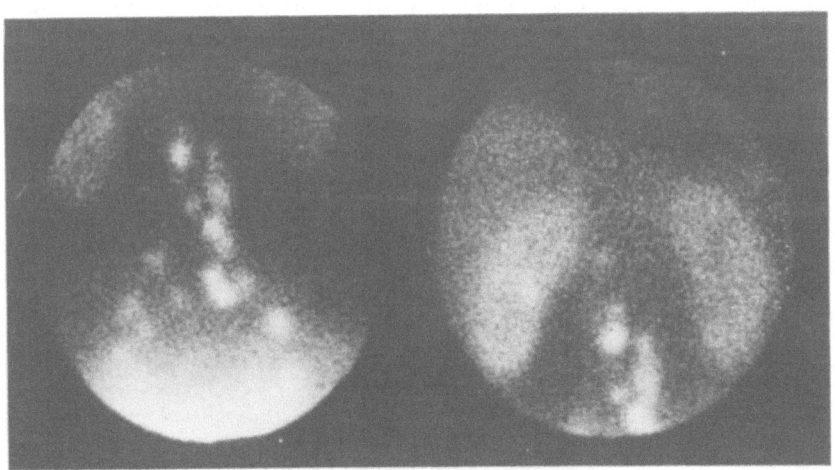

Figure 26-1. Normal study. Internal, common, and paraaortic
nodes seen on the anterior view (left) to the level of the
renal hilum bilaterally (right).

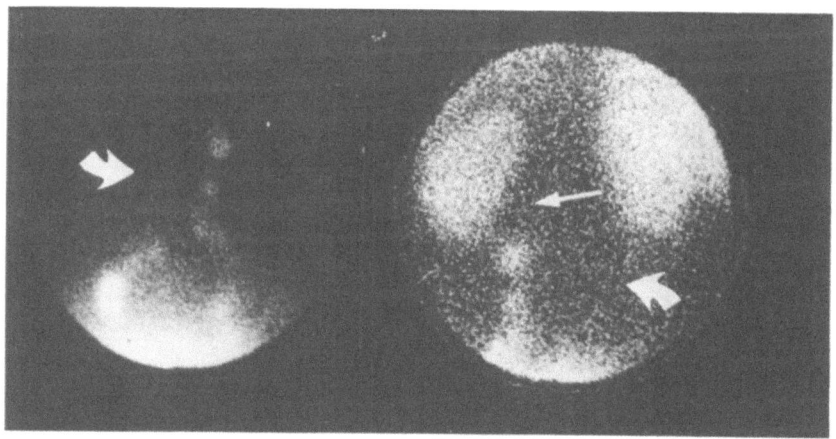

Figure 26-2.  Anterior view (left) shows incomplete filling of
the right common iliac nodes (curved arrow) and filling of
left para-aortics to level of lower pole of kidney.  On the
posterior view of the kidneys (right), the para-aortics are
seen to fill only to the lower pole of the left kidney
(straight arrow).  Pathology revealed large tumor-filled node
at this level and microscopic infiltration of entire non-
visualized right-sided para-aortic chain.


TABLE 26-2

RESULTS OF CORROBORATIVE FINDINGS IN 32 PATIENTS
UNDERGOING ILIOPELVIC LYMPHOSCINTIGRAPHY (10)

SURGICOPATHOLOGY

|          |     | +    | -    |
|----------|-----|------|------|
|          | +   | .70  | .08  |
| Scan     |     |      |      |
|          | -   | .30  | .92  |
| No. Pts. |     | 20   | 12   |

In her initial report, Ege further defined 32 patients who underwent lymphoscintigraphic studies and had corroborative surgicopathologic findings (Table 26-2). An analysis of the results in those patients showed a sensitivity of 70% (a positive scan result in the presence of pathologically proven abnormal lymph nodes), and a specificity of 92% (a negative scan result in a patient with normal nodes).

Over the past two years, in a collaborative study between the Sidney Farber Cancer Institute and the Brigham and Women's Hospital, we have had the opportunity to perform iliopelvic lymphoscintigraphy in 21 patients presenting with testicular carcinoma (15 non-seminoma, six seminoma) (13). In the 15 non-seminoma patients, staging lymphadenectomies revealed a sensitivity of 89% and a specificity of 83%. Although staging lymphadenectomies were not performed in the six seminoma patients, the results of a number of other non-invasive radiologic studies (lymphangiography, computed tomography, and ultrasound) were available (Table 26-3). This latter correlation showed good agreement between the findings on iliopelvic lymphoscintiscans and the results of at least two of three other radiologic studies.

TABLE 26-3

SCAN RESULTS IN SIX SEMINOMA PATIENTS AS CORRELATED WITH
RESULTS OF OTHER RADIOLOGIC TESTS (13)

| PATIENT | IPLS | LAG | CT | US |
|---------|------|-----|----|----|
| 1 | − | − | − | 0 |
| 2 | − | − | − | − |
| 3 | − | − | 0 | 0 |
| 4 | + | + | + | − |
| 5 | + | 0 | + | + |
| 6 | + | − | + | + |

| | | |
|------|---|---------------------------|
| IPLS | = | Iliopelvic Lymphoscintigraphy |
| LAG | = | Contrast Lymphangiography |
| CT | = | Computerized Tomography |
| US | = | Ultrasound |
| 0 | = | Test Not Performed |
| + | = | Positive |
| − | = | Negative |

There are numerous advantages for implementing iliopelvic
lymphoscintigraphy in the evaluation of lymphatic integrity in
patients with pelvic malignancy.  The technique provides a
method for rapid, non-invasive access to pelvic lymphatics.
Additionally, it is physiologic since volumes on the order of
0.2 ml of radiocolloid in normal saline are being administered.

The procedure appears to offer "functional" information of
lymph node integrity rather than anatomic data.  In a number
of our patients, the presence of microscopic nodal metastases
was sufficient to alter radiocolloid uptake.  Of importance,
in these patients, CT studies and the observation of the
surgeon at the time of lymphadenectomy suggested that the
nodes were normal.

Another distinct advantage is the routine recognition of
six lymph node groups.  These groups are outlined in Table
26-4.  Of clinical significance, the internal iliac nodes are
visualized on 98% of the iliopelvic lymphoscintiscans.
Bipedal injections of oily contrast for lymphangiography will
not consistently allow this level of accurate delineation for
this group of nodes.

In our experience, this non-invasive radionuclide technique appears to offer improved accuracy in the clinical
staging of pelvic malignancies and the ability to indivi-
dualize patient management in a variety of pelvic neoplasms.

TABLE 26-4

LYMPH NODE GROUPS IDENTIFIED DURING ILIOPELVIC
LYMPHOSCINTIGRAPHY IN 58 PATIENTS (10)

| NODAL GROUP | PERCENT |
|---|---|
| Para-aortic | 100 |
| Pre-sacral | 70 |
| Common Iliac | 100 |
| External Iliac | 36 |
| Internal Iliac | 98 |
| Para-rectal | 45 |

SELECTED REFERENCES

1. Wood, D.A., et al.: Staging of cancer of the colon and cancer of the rectum. Cancer 43:961, 1979.

2. Schmidt, J.D. and Weinstein, H.: Pitfalls in clinical staging of bladder tumors. Urol. Clin. North. Am. 3:107, 1976.

3. Grossman, I.C., et al.: Staging pelvic lymphadenectomy for carcinoma of the prostate: review of 91 cases. J. Urol. 124:632, 1980.

4. Dunnick, N.R. and Javadpour, N.: Value of CT and lymphography: distinguishing retroperitoneal metastases from non-seminomatous testicular tumors. Am. J. Roent. 136:1093, 1981.

5. Thomas, J.L., Bernardino, M.E. and Bracken, R.B.: Staging of testicular carcinoma: comparison of CT and lymphography. Am. J. Roent. 137:991, 1981.

6. Richie, J.P., Garnick, M.B. and Finberg, H.: Computed tomography: how accurate for abdominal staging of testis tumors? J. Urol. 127:715, 1982.

7. Matsuo, S.: Studies on the metastasis of breast cancer to lymph nodes II. Diagnosis of metastasis to internal mammary nodes using radiocolloid. Acta. Med. Okayama. 28:361, 1974.

8. Osborne, M.P., et al.: The preoperative detection of internal mammary lymph node metastases in breast cancer. Br. J. Surg. 66:813, 1979.

9. Black, R.B., et al.: Prediction of axillary metastasis in breast cancer by lymphoscintigraphy. Lancet 2:15, 1980.

10. Ege, G.N. and Cummings, B.J.: Interstitial radiocolloid iliopelvic lymphoscintigraphy: technique, anatomy, and clinical application. Int. J. Radiat. Oncol. 6:1483, 1980.

11. Ege, G.N.: Augmented iliopelvic lymphoscintigraphy: application in the management of genitourinary malignancy. J. Urol. 127:265, 1982.

228                                           CHAPTER 26

12. Enqvist, I.F. and Block, I.R.:  Rectal cancer in the
    female:  selection of proper operation based upon anatomic
    studies of rectal lymphatics.  Prog. Clin. Cancer 2:73,
    1966.

13. Kaplan, W.D., Garnick, M.B., and Richie, J.P.:  Iliopelvic
    radionuclide lymphoscintigraphy in patients with
    testicular cancer.  Radiology, In Press, 1983.

14. Herman, P.G., et al.:  Roentgen anatomy of the
    ilio-pelvic-aorta lymph system.  Radiology 80:182, 1963.

15. Chiappa S, et al.:  Combined testicular and foot
    lymphangiography in testicular carcinomas.  Surg. Gynec.
    Obstet. 123:10, 1966.

CHAPTER 27

A NEW MARKER FOR THE DETECTION OF TRANSITIONAL CELL CARCINOMA

Bruce R. Zetter

Transitional cell carcinoma of the bladder is a form of malignant lesion for which the rate of recurrence following surgical intervention is particularly high. At present, the detection and management of these recurrent tumors depends largely on periodic cystoscopy of individuals with a history of bladder cancer. The efficacy of this practice depends on patient compliance to an invasive diagnostic procedure as well as on the limits of the technique to detect small tumor foci. A second widely used procedure involves cytological examination of tumor cells shed into the urine. This method is generally accurate for high grade tumors but has given rise to as much as 50% false positives when used for the detection of recurrent bladder tumors. False positive results have also been reported for cytological screening in individuals undergoing radiation therapy or intravesical chemotherapy.

Clearly there is room for improvement in the detection of bladder carcinoma both for individuals with a history of the disease and for those at high risk due to environmental exposure to carcinogens. Indeed, detection of urothelial tumors should be facilitated by the direct release of tumor products into the urine without prior processing in the bloodstream or kidney. The rapid developments in this field in the past few years have resulted in the publication of several new markers or screening techniques for bladder tumors. Rather than discussing the relative advantages and disadvantages of each new marker, I would like, in this paper, to share our experiences in the development of one potential new screening protocol for the detection of transitional cell carcinoma of the bladder.

To search for a diagnostic marker in human urine, one must adopt either of two basic strategies. The first is to non-selectively try to detect any molecule that is present in the urine of tumor patients but missing in control urine. This approach has been used with varying degrees of success for enzymes, amino acids, polyamines, fibrinopeptides and fibronectin along with a large variety of antigens most of which have yet to be structurally or functionally identified. This approach generally requires a sensitive biochemical assay or immunological screening protocol performed on a large number of samples. A second approach is to select a biological parameter known to be expressed by the tumor in vivo and to screen urine for evidence of this specific tumor activity. This second approach will generally rely on a bioassay to detect the biological activity in the urine sample.

In the present study, we have used the tumor's ability to attract new blood vessels as a model for the development of a screening protocol. This work derived from initial studies by Chodak et al. who showed that biopsy specimens from patients with transitional cell carcinoma (TCC) stimulated the directional growth of new capillaries when implanted into rabbit corneas. Since these tumor fragments were able to release a substance that could diffuse through the avascular corneal tissue to stimulate the growth of limbal blood vessels, it seemed reasonable to ask whether transitional cell tumors in situ would secrete detectable amounts of the same material into the urine. We therefore decided to collect urine from bladder tumor patients before and after transurethral resection of the tumor in order to determine whether the presence of capillary-stimulating (angiogenic) activity would be a useful marker for the presence of new or recurrent TCC.

The bioassay that we chose for the study was based on the observation by Ausprunk and Folkman that migration of capillary endothelial cells is required for the directional growth of new blood vessels toward a tumor stimulus. Since a sensitive, quantitative assay for endothelial cell migration had recently been developed, we were able to monitor human urine to determine levels of endothelial cell migration-stimulating activity. The assay entails placing cultured capillary endothelial cells onto surfaces that have been uniformily coated with a film of fine particles such as latex beads or colloidal gold. The endothelial cells phagocytize the particles they encounter and, if the cells are stimulated

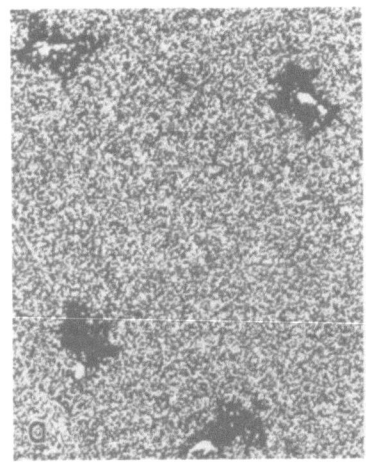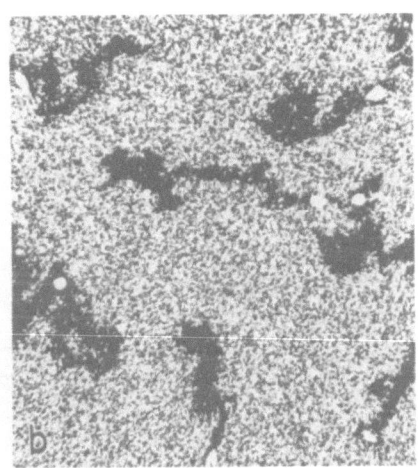

Figure 27-1.  Phagokinetic tracks made by capillary endothelial cells moving across gold-coated coverslips in the absence
(a) or presence (b) of tumor-derived migration factors.

to migrate, they leave empty tracks that serve as a permanent
record of their movement (Fig. 27-1).  For each sample, we
routinely measure the area of 100 of these "phagokinetic
tracks" and use the mean track area as a measure of the induced endothelial cell motility.

    The results to date have been quite encouraging.  Multiple
samples of concentrated, dialyzed urine from 21 patients with
gross TCC all had significant activity in the endothelial cell
migration assay (mean increase in track area = 42% above
unstimulated control) (Fig. 27-2).  The amount of activity in
a given patient's urine was directly proportional to the size
of that patient's tumor but bore no relation to tumor grade.
However, even patients with small tumors (0.5 cm diameter) had
significant levels of migration-stimulating activity in their
urine.  Activities in the urine of 3 different control groups
were reduced relative to the patients with TCC.  Samples from
22 patients with no known disease had a mean activity of only
16% (increase relative to control) whereas 42 patients with
non-malignant disease including pyelonephritis, prostatitis,
cystitis, urinary traact infections, urethral stricture and
others as depicted in Table 27-1 had mean activity of only
10.0%.  Furthermore, urine from patients with a recent or
prior history of bladder carcinoma also had reduced activity

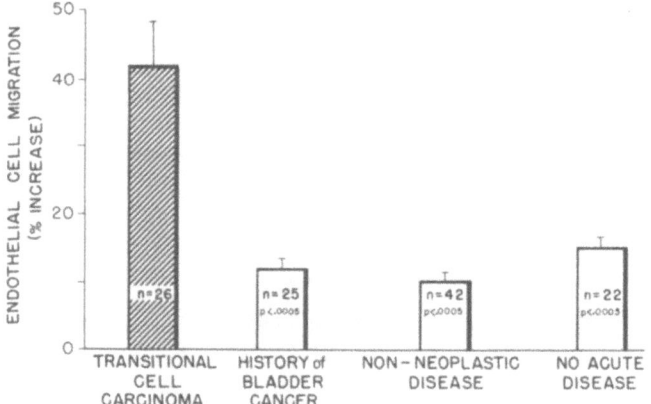

Figure 27-2. Mean endothelial cell migration activity in four
groups of patients. Mean activity (+ S.E.M.) is shown for 26
samples from 21 patients with gross transitional cell carcinoma of the bladder or ureter, 25 samples from 21 patients
with a history of bladder cancer but no tumor present at the
time of cystoscopy, 42 samples from 42 patients with
non-neoplastic disease, and 22 samples from 22 healthy
volunteers.


(12% over control).

    In order to determine whether tumor removal would cause a
decrease in the amount of migration-stimulating activity in
the urine, we tested urine samples collected from 10 patients
both immediately before and 3-6 days after TUR. In every
case, the levels of activity fell markedly after surgery
(Table 27-2). The mean level of activity for the samples
collected preoperatively was 42.6% compared with 10.0% for the
postoperative samples. The patients chosen for this study had
no significant changes in medication regimen in the time
between the first and second samplings.

    The reduction in urinary endothelial cell migration
activity following tumor removal allowed us to ask whether a
recurrent tumor would result in a recurrent elevation of
migration activity in the urine. Because patients with a
history of TCC undergo periodic cystoscopic examinations, we
were able to compare our migration assay results with the
results of the cystoscopic examinations. Four of the patients

Table 27-1.   Endothelial Cell Migration-Stimulating Activity
in Human Urine.

| Diagnosis | No. Samples | Cell Migration (Mean % Inc + SEM) |
|---|---|---|
| Preoperative transitional cell CA | 26 | 42 ± 6 |
| Postoperative transitional cell CA | 11 | 9 ± 2 |
| Past history of transitional cell CA | 14 | 15 ± 2 |
| Carcinoma of the prostate | 8 | 7 ± 2 |
| Preoperative squamous cell CA (bladder) | 2 | 7 ± 3 |
| Pyelonephritis | 2 | 18 ± 2 |
| Prostatitis | 5 | 11 ± 3 |
| Benign prostatic hypertrophy | 3 | 15 ± 4 |
| Genitourinary infections | 8 | 7 ± 3 |
| Other benign urological diseases | 12 | 11 ± 3 |
| Colitis | 3 | 8 ± 4 |
| Crohn's disease | 4 | 8 ± 3 |
| Other benign diseases | 5 | 11 ± 2 |
| Healthy volunteers | 22 | 16 ± 2 |

in the group that had been tested pre- and postoperatively
were followed for 3-12 months after surgery.  In one of these
patients, there has been no recurrence of new tumor growth and
no increase in the urinary migration-stimulating activity over
a nine-month period.  The three other patients, however, had
tumors grossly evident by cystoscopy between 3 and 6 months
following surgery.  For each of these patients, the level of
migration-stimulating activity found in the urine was markedly
elevated at the time that new tumor was detected.  It should
be noted that the individuals performing the migration assays
had no knowledge of the diagnosis at the time they tested any

Table 27-2.  Evaluation of Migration-Stimulating Activity
Prior to and after Resection of Bladder Tumors.

| Patient No. | Migration Activity (% of Increase) | |
| --- | --- | --- |
| | Preoperative | Postoperative |
| 1 (First Hosp.) | 59 | 7 |
| (Second Hosp.) | 38 | 17 |
| 2 | 40 | 15 |
| 4 | 25 | 6 |
| 5 | 34 | 6 |
| 6 | 21 | 11 |
| 7 | 39 | 10 |
| 8 | 50 | 0 |
| 9 | 94 | 20 |
| 10 | 23 | 6 |
| 13 | 38 | 8 |
| Mean + S.E.M. | $42 \pm 6$ | $10 \pm 2$ |

of the specimens.

Several other patients with a long-term history of bladder
carcinoma are currently being followed with this new assay.
In 2 of these cases, new or recurrent tumors have been simultaneously detected by an increase in migration activity and by
cystoscopic examination.  In two other cases, however, we have
detected an increase in migration-stimulating activity with no
concomitant cystoscopically evident tumor.  One of these
patients subsequently developed grossly evident new tumor
growth some months after the elevated migration activity was
first observed.  Since small malignant tumors and even certain
forms of preneoplastic lesion have been found to release
angiogenesis factors, we consider it possible that the expression of this activity may precede the growth of recurrent
bladder tumor to visible dimensions.  If reproducible, this
result may indicate an increased sensitivity on the part of
this assay to detect small, low grade tumors that might be
missed by other procedures.

To date, we have not experienced any false negative
results from patients with verified TCC but we have seen 2
false positives.  Both were seen in healthy young (under 30
years) women with no evidence of benign or malignant

urological disease.  On subsequent testings, neither had
elevated activity.  We do not presently understand the meaning
of these 2 results but it should be noted that neovascular-
ization is an important component of the female reproductive
cycle and that angiogenesis factors involved in this process
have already been reported.  It is therefore conceivable that
such factors could make their way into the urine of normal
women.  However, since this activity was seen in only 2 of 52
women tested and since urothelial tumors most commonly occur
in men or in post-menopausal women, this phenomenon may not
seriously impair the diagnostic efficacy of the assay.

Our success with the use of urinary endothelial cell
migration-stimulating activity as a marker for new and
recurrent transitional cell carcinoma confirms that angiogenesis activity is a useful marker for the detection of
certain bladder tumors.  Similar migration-stimulating
activity has also been found in the aqueous humor of patients
with retinoblatoma or choroidal melanoma as well as in the
cerebrospinal fluid of patients with meningioma.  I do not
wish to suggest that the assay in its present form will be the
most effective way to routinely detect bladder carcinoma,
although it may be a useful adjunct to cystoscopy for individuals at high risk.  The current protocol, however, requires
expensive image analysis equipment as well as expertise in the
cell culture of capillary endothelial cells that are beyond
the scope of most hospital laboratories.  Our present emphasis
is on the purification of the migration-stimulating factor
from TCC and the eventual production of a monoclonal antibody
to this factor for use in radioimmunoassay.  The development
of these tools may lead to sensitive and widely used screening
techniques.

SELECTED REFERENCES

1.  Lessing, J.A.:  Bladder cancer: Early diagnosis and
    evaluation of biologic potential.  A review of newer
    methods.  J. Urol. 120: 1, 1978.

2.  McGregor, R.F., et al.:  Urinary amino acid excretion.
    Urol. 9:538, 1977.

3.  Sanford, E.J., et al.:  Preliminary evaluation of urinary
    polyamines in GU malignancy.  J. Urol. 113:218, 1975.

4. Wejsman, C., et al.: Evaluation of biological markers in bladder cancer. J. Urol. 114:879, 1975.

5. Gozzo, J.J., et al.: Detection of tumor associated antigens in urine from patients with bladder cancer. J. Urol. 124:804, 1980.

6. Gullino, P.: Angiogenesis and Neoplasia. N. Engl. J. Med. 305:884, 1981.

7. Chodak, G.W., et al.: Angiogenic activity as a marker of bladder lesions. Ann Surg. 192:762, 1980.

8. Zetter, B.R. Migration of capillary endothelial cells is stimulated by tumor-derived factors. Nature 285:41, 1980.

9. Chodak, G.W., Scheiner, C.J., Zetter, B.R.: Urine from patient with transitional cell carcinoma stimulates migration of capillary endothelial cells. N. Engl. J. Med. 305:869, 1981.

10. Tapper, D., et. al.: Angiogenesis capacity as a diagnostic marker for human eye tumors. Surgery 86:36, 1979.

CHAPTER 28

IN VITRO CLONOGENIC CHEMOSENSITIVITY ASSAY IN UROLOGIC TUMORS

Donald G. Skinner

The in vitro clonogenic chemosensitivity test, utilizing
soft agar cultural media, has been used in the laboratory
since March 1980.  Urologic tumor specimens obtained at the
time of surgery from 96 patients have been tested against a
panel of up to 20 chemotherapeutic agents (Table 28-1).
Growth of 21 of 22 renal cancers, 18 of 19 urothelial cancers,
and 20 of 24 testicular cancers has been achieved.  Successful
chemosensitivity testing has also been accomplished on bladder
lavage specimens (8 of 14) with close correspondence to
results obtained from surgical specimens, but the number of
cells obtained has restricted the number of drugs tested.  The
cloning efficiency has been comparable for all histologic
types and for primary, nodal, metastatic and lavage
specimens.  Comparative evaluation of the sensitivity profile
shows a tendency for renal cell carcinoma to be more resistant
than either transitional cell carcinoma or testicular cancer,
but less than would be anticipated by clinical experience.

The heterogeneity of response to a specific drug of histologically identical tumor derived from different patients
would suggest that current adjuvant chemotherapy trials using
single drug protocols are less than optimal and that future
trials should incorporate in vitro chemosensitivity testing
and combination therapy.

Without question cancer chemotherapy has improved substantially within the past decade due, in part, to the
development of better drugs and a concept of earlier
aggressive treatment and use of combination therapy.

237

TABLE 28-1.   Source of specimens of urologic malignancies
submitted for in vitro clonogenic chemosensitivity test.  Successful growth indicated
according to site and source (T = primary tumor;
N = regional node; M = metastatic site).

| Site | T | N | M | Lavage | Urine | All | |
|------|---|---|---|--------|-------|-----|---|
|      |   |   |   | Specimen Source | | | |
| Prostate | 1/1 | 4/5 | 2/2 | | | 7/8 | (88%) |
| Bladder | 9/10 | 4/4 | 5/5 | 6/14 | 3/9 | 27/42 | (64%) |
| Testis | 5/6 | 6/7 | 9/11 | | | 20/24 | (83%) |
| Kidney | 14/15 | 3/3 | 4/4 | | | 21/22 | (95%) |

Nonetheless, selection of effective drugs for individual
patients remains a trial and error procedure.  Until now
predictive techniques similar to culture and sensitivity
assay used for management of infections have not been
available.  Early clinical trials suggest that in vitro
chemosensitivity testing may make predictive cancer therapy
feasible.

  While development of this assay may facilitate
drug selection for cancer chemotherapy, clinicians should
recognize the limitation of this procedure.  There remain
problems which limit its usefulness.  The following constraints must be kept in mind:
     (1)   There are factors other than in vitro
sensitivity that contribute to a probability of achieving
response to drug treatment.  Among these factors are
patient ability to withstand treatment, in vivo tumor
kinetics, and access of drug to tumor as well as other
properties of cancer in man that have not been identified.
     (2)   The success of the assay is only as good as
the material it is provided.  Tumor samples must be viable,
properly selected, and in sufficient quantity (5 gm.
minimum) to provide greater than $2 \times 10^7$ cells.
     (3)   Cells from some tumors simply will not grow
in agar.
     (4)   The plating efficiency or number of
colonies in some cases will not be sufficient to allow
testing of a sufficient number of drugs.
     (5)   The tumor may grow well in the assay but no
effective drugs may be identified.

To illustrate these limitations vonHoff has prospectively studied 110 patients with colon, breast or head and neck tumors. All patients had measurable metastatic disease and were managed by either standard chemotherapy methods or according to chemosensitivity test when sensitive drugs were identified. Patients were assigned to four groups:  Group A – no development of tumor colonies; Group B – tumor growth but insufficient colonies to allow drug testing; Group C – good tumor growth but no drugs killing more than 50% colonies; Group D – good colony growth and sensitive drugs. Only 25 of the 110 patients entered in this protocol fit into the Group D category and were treated by selective single agent chemotherapy. The other 85 patients received the traditional chemotherapy with objective response rate of less than 15% as defined by greater than 50% reduction of measurable disease. None of the patients in whom tumor resistance was predicted by the assay showed a clinical response. The 25 patients treated selectively, however, enjoyed a 44% objective response rate. So far there has been no report of clinical trials using combination therapy selected by the chemosensitivity assay. This data implies that the chemosensitivity assay currently has limitations in clinical applicability to many patients until more effective anti–cancer agents are developed, but that it is reliable in predicting resistance, thus obviating the need to subject patients to toxic drugs without reasonable expectation of benefit.

The test may have its most important role in the surgical adjuvant setting for cancers with high preponderance of micrometastases. If the bioassay results predict utility of treatment, early aggressive prophylactic therapy could be promptly initiated before evidence of overt relapse. We currently have initiated prospective clinical trials of adjuvant chemotherapy selected by the in vitro assay for patients with transitional cell carcinoma of the bladder following cystectomy and for patients with advanced renal cell carcinoma following nephrectomy.

In conclusion, preliminary data reveals that the in vitro clonogenic stem cell assay is an important new tool that should allow tailoring of individual chemotherapy and identification of useful agents, both traditional and experimental, that may have a major impact on future chemotherapy trials.

240                                                        CHAPTER 28

SUGGESTED REFERENCES

1. Hamburger, A.W. and Salmon, S.E.:  Primary bioassay of human tumor stem cells.  Science 197:401, 1977

2. Hamburger, A.W., et al.:  Direct cloning of human ovarian carcinoma cells in agar.  Cancer Res. 38:3438, 1978.

3. Daniels, J.R., et al.:  Chemosensitivity of human neoplasms utilizing in vitro clone formation.  Experience at the University of Southern California-Los Angeles County Medical Center.  Submitted for publication, Cancer Res., 1981.

4. Salmon, S.E. and Buick, R.N.:  Preparation of permanent slides of intact soft-agar colony cultures of hematopoietin and tumor stem cells.  Cancer Res., 39:1133, 1979.

5. Sarosdy, M.F., et al.:  Clonogenic assay and in vitro chemosensitivity testing of human urologic malignancies.  Cancer 50:1332, 1982.

6. vonHoff, D.D. and Johnson, G.E.:  Secretion of tumor markers in the human tumor stem cell assay system.  Proc. Am. Assoc. Cancer Res. 22:51, 1979.

7. vonHoff, D.D.:  New leads from the laboratory for testing testicular cancer.  In:  VanOostrom, A.T., Muggia, F.M. and Cleton, F.J., eds. Therapeutic Progress in Ovarian Cancer, Testicular Cancer and the Sarcomas.  Amsterdam: Leiden University Press, 1980, p. 225.

8. Puck, T.T., Marcus, P.I. and Ciecura, S.J.:  Clonal growth of mammalian cells in vitro.  J. Exp. Med., 103:273, 1955.

9. McAllister, R., Reed, G. and Huebower, R.J.:  Colonial growth in agar of cells derived from adenovirus-induced hamster tissue.  J. Clin. Cancer Inst. 39:43, 1967.

10. McAllister, R. and Reed, G.:  Colonial growth in agar of cells derived from neoplastic and non-neoplastic tissue of children.  Pediatric Res. 2:356, 1968.

11. Salmon, S.E., Soehnlen, B. and Alberts, D.S.:  New drugs in ovarian cancer:  In vitro phase II screening with the

human tissue stem cell assay. In: VanOostrom, A.T., Muggia, F. and Cleton, F.J., eds. Therapeutic Progress in Ovarian Cancer, Testicular Cancer and the Sarcomas. Amsterdam: Leiden University Press, 1980, p. 113.

CHAPTER 29

CARCINOMA OF THE ADRENAL CORTEX


Jerome P. Richie




Adrenal cortical carcinomas are rare tumors that may arise
from any one of the layers of the adrenal cortex. Tumors are
classified as "functioning", if cortical steroids in excess
are produced, or "non-functioning" when no clinical evidence
exists of endocrine derangement. Non-functioning tumors are
considerably rarer than functioning tumors, with only 178
reported cases up to 1974. The incidence is approximately
2/million population/year. The majority of patients are
female, and the mean age at diagnosis is in the 4th decade.
Females may be diagnosed more commonly and at an earlier age
because of virilization secondary to functioning adrenal
tumors.

Multiple manifestations may be noted in patients with
adrenal cortical neoplasms - Cushing's syndrome, the adrenogenital syndrome, precocious puberty, or hyperaldosteronism.
In prepubertal females, virilization after birth is most
commonly caused by adrenal carcinoma. Progressive virilization after normal appearing external genitalia at birth is
suggestive of adrenal neoplasm. In adult females, masculine
changes occur with early hirsutism and temporal balding.
Amenorrhea is common and masculine changes in the muscular
habitus and voice may ensue. A mixed syndrome of
adrenogenital syndrome and Cushing's syndrome in an adult
female is strongly suggestive of adrenal cortical carcinoma.

Feminization in the adult male may be the result of an
estrogen-producing tumor. Symptoms may be gynecomastia,
testicular atrophy, impotency, obesity, and oligospermia.

243

Non-functioning adrenal cortical neoplasms do not give
rise to major endocrine symptoms; consequently, these tumors
are usually discovered only after they have grown to substantial size or metastasized. The tumor may remain asymptomatic
and present as a large abdominal mass. Hemorrhage and
necrosis may produce pain, backache, or fever.


ENDOCRINE EVALUATION

With a suspected adrenal cortical tumor, appropriate
determinations of plasma and urinary steroid levels with
stimulation and suppression may be obtained. However,
endocrine evaluation should be expeditious so as not to unduly
delay appropriate therapy. Patients with adrenal cancer
commonly excrete large amounts of urinary 17-ketosteroids,
regardless of the clinical symptomatology. Urinary free
cortisol and 17-hydroxycorticoids may also be elevated.

Feminizing adrenal tumors in males secrete increased
amounts of androstenedione which is converted into estrogens
by the liver. Therefore, serum and urinary estrogen levels
are increased. Adrenal androgen is also increased, as
evidenced by elevated urinary 17-ketosteroids.

Non-functioning adrenal cortical carcinomas may be capable
of forming excess precursor steroids. Levels of urinary
17-ketosteroids and 17-hydroxysteroids are normal. However,
some of these patients will demonstrate increased levels of
hormonally inactive precursors, such as metabolities of
pregnenolone.


RADIOLOGIC DIAGNOSIS

Calcification in the adrenal area should be considered
suspicious of adrenal neoplasm. Excretory urography will help
determine whether a lesion arises from the kidney or from the
adrenal. With adrenal carcinoma, the kidney is often dis-
placed downward without distortion of the calyceal system,
retaining the parallel nature of the long axis of the kidney
and of the calyces.

Controversy exists over the efficacy of ultrasound, CT
scan, arteriography, and venography in the diagnosis of
adrenal lesions. Sonography may be effective but is very

operator-dependent. CT scan has proved highly accurate and
less dependent upon skill of interpretation and has become the
procedure of choice for demonstration of adrenal lesions.
Stewart and associates stated that any lesion larger than 1
cm. could be delineated accurately. CT scan not only provides
the extent and location of adrenal tumors and normal adrenal
glands but also provides information about the precise
relationship of the tumor to adjacent organs.

Arteriography and selective arteriography remain valuable
for differentiation of adrenal from upper pole renal neoplasms. Adrenal venography is indicated if an IVP with
tomography and the CT scan do not pinpoint a tumor, since
venography can reveal lesions less than 1 cm. in diameter. In
addition, the potential of drawing venous samples for analysis
is available. Adrenal venography does carry some morbidity,
especially intra adrenal hemorrhage and adrenal insufficiency.

Functional radionuclide scans, using iodinated choles-
terol, appear to be promising for diagnosis and detection of
metastatic lesions. The use of $^{131}$I-19-iodocholesterol as a
scanning agent has been described. Recently, $^{131}$I-6-beta-
iodomethyl-19-norcholesterol has been shown to achieve
superior concentration in adrenal tissue.


STAGING

Staging is important from both a therapeutic and
prognostic aspect. A staging system, including a TNM system,
is outlined in Table 29-1. Most male patients are seen with
advanced stage tumors, whereas females have a more even
distribution of stage. In general, younger patients tend to
have lower stage tumors as well.


OPERATIVE TREATMENT

Radical excision with wide exposure remains the primary
treatment for all adrenal tumors. Usually the best approach
is via the thoracoabdominal approach on the ipsilateral side.
This provides access to the tumor, the regional lymph nodes,
and adjacent vital structures. Adrenal carcinomas tend to be
quite large, the average diameter being 10.1 cm. with a range
of 2.5-21 cm. En bloc dissection may require extrafascial
dissection, nephrectomy, splenectomy, or partial pancreat-

Table 29-1.  Staging of Adrenocortical Tumors

| Stage | Size of primary | Local Nodes/Invasion | Metastases | TNM |
|---|---|---|---|---|
| 1 | less 5 cm | - | - | - | T1NOMO |
| 2 | over 5 cm | - | - | - | T2NOMO |
| 3 | Any size | - | + | - | T3NOMO |
|  |  | + | - | - | T1-2N1MO |
|  |  | + | + | - | T3N1MO |
| 4 | Any size |  |  | + | M1 |

ectomy.  Proper preoperative preparation and surgical exposure
can lead to potential cure even in very large masses.
However, adequate resection is imperative.

ADJUVANT AND ADVANCED THERAPY

Chemotherapy has generally been disappointing.  Ortho para
DDD (Mitotane) has been described for the treatment of adrenal
cortical carcinomas.  Hutter and Kayhoe reported on 138
patients treated with this agent and found the mean duration
of steroid response to be five months.  An overall 45% clinical response has been reported.  The duration of life from
onset of treatment was 8.4 months, demonstrating the dismal
survival with this tumor.

The dosage of ortho para DDD is 2 to 6 g per day in
divided doses.  Toxic side effects, predominantly involving
the GI tract and neuromuscular system, are seen in 90% of
patients.  A recent study has reported reduced incidence of GI
discomfort when cellulose acetylphthalate has been added.
This allows passage of the ortho para DDD through the stomach
and may account for the diminished gastrointestinal side
effects seen with the addition of this agent.

A rare "cure" has been reported with chemotherapy using
ortho para DDD.  However, the overall poor response in
advanced disease stresses the need for phase II studies and
combined collaborative chemotherapy treatment studies.

The role of radiation therapy in the management of adrenal
cortical carcinoma has been infrequently documented.  Most

authors conclude that radiation therapy has little or no effect on the primary adrenal tumor or its metastases. Radiation therapy may be useful for palliation from bony metastases.

Some preliminary evidence has documented activity for single agent cis-platinum in the management of patients with advanced disease.

SUGGESTED REFERENCES

1.  Becker, D. and Schumacher, O.P.: O,P¹ DDD therapy in invasive adrenocortical carcinoma. Ann. Int. Med. 82:677, 1975.

2.  Bennett, A.H., Harrison, J.H. and Thorn, G.W.: Neoplasms of the adrenal gland. J. Urol. 106:607, 1971.

3.  Fritzsche, P., Andersen, C., and Cahill, P.: Vascular specificity in differentiating adrenal carcinoma from renal cell carcinoma. Radiology 125:113, 1977.

4.  Hajjar, R.A., Hickey, R.C. and Samaan, N.A.: Adrenal cortical carcinoma. Cancer 35:549, 1975.

5.  Hutter, A.M., Jr. and Kayhoe, D.E.: Adrenal cortical carcinoma: Clinical features of 138 patients. Am. J. Med. 41:581, 1966.

6.  Richie, J.P. and Gittes, R.F.: Carcinoma of the adrenal cortex. Cancer 45:1957, 1980.

7.  Sample, W.F.: Adrenal ultrasonography. Radiology 127:461, 1978.

8.  Stewart, B.H., et al.: Urologic applications of computerized axial tomography: A preliminary report. J. Urol. 120:660, 1978.

9.  Sullivan, M., Boileau, M. and Hodges, C.V.: Adrenal cortical carcinoma. J. Urol. 120:660, 1978.

CHAPTER 30A

CARCINOMA OF THE PENIS

Willet F. Whitmore, III

I. PENILE LESIONS

A. Benign - may be mistaken for carcinoma
   - condyloma acuminata
   - giant condyloma
   - pseudo-epitheliomatous hyperplasia

B. Premalignant
   - Uncategorized dysplasias
   - Erythroplasia of Queyrat (10% develop invasive cancer)

C. Malignant
   - Bowen's disease = squamous cell CIS
     1. 5% develop invasive lesion
     2. 40% develop other premalignant or malignant skin lesion
     3. 25% develop primary visceral carcinoma
   - Verrucous carcinoma - (low metastatic potential)
   - Squamous cell carcinoma (invasive)

II. SQUAMOUS CELL CARCINOMA

A. In the U.S.
   - 0.5% of all male malignancies
   - age range 20-90 years
   - 80% of patients over age 50

B. Epidemiology
   - cause unknown
   - circumcision preventive

C. Histology
   - well to moderately well differentiated
   - little bearing on prognosis

D. Natural history -- Orderly systematic progression
   1. Begins as lesion on the penile skin
   2. Invades locally and ulcerates -- infection
   3. Metastasizes regionally to the inguinal lymph
      nodes
   4. Invades locally in the groin causing ulceration,
      infection and erosion into vessels and bone
   5. Metastases to pelvic lymph nodes occur as groin
      involvement progresses.
   6. Systemic blood born metastases occur late - lung
      most common site.

E. Presentation (most --- least common)
   - penile mass
   - ulcerating lesion
   - penile pain or discharge
   - lymphadenopathy

F. Staging Classification (Jackson)
   Stage I  =  tumor limited to glans penis and/or
               foreskin
   Stage II = tumor invasive into the corpora without
               nodal or distant metastases
   Stage III= tumor with regional lymphatic metastases
   Stage IV = inoperable regional disease and/or
               distant metastases

G. Clinical Staging
   1. Workup:
      a. physical examination
      b. chest x-ray
      c. IVP
      d. lymphangiogram - no value
      e. CT scan - ? value
      f. sentinel lymph node biopsy (?)
   2. Accuracy - imprecise
      Stage I
      Stage II  False positive 20%

Stage III False negative 40%
(infection/inflammation)
(probably less because of potential misses in
histologic sampling)

H. Paraneoplastic Syndrome
1. associated hypercalcemia without osseous mets
   most common (a function of tumor volume that will
   resolve with removal of tumor mass)

I. Primary Lesion    Treatment Recommendations and
   Rationale:
   1. Stage I
      a. local resection (with margins nagative
         recurrence less than 10%)
      b. partial amputation (2 cm. margin)
      c. irradiation therapy (dose over 5000R)
         - 25% stricture
         - 10% penile necrosis
         - 10-50% risk of recurrence
      d. chemotherapy + systemic or topical
         ? combination with irradiation therapy
   2. Stage II, III, IV
      a. partial or total amputation
      b. radiotherapy of no value when normal anatomy
         destroyed by tumor
      c. chemotherapy ?

J. Regional Metastases - Treatment recommendations and
   rationale

   Stages I and II

   1. Background data
      a. over 80% of patients with Stage I and less
         than 80% with Stage II disease will be cured
         by treatment of the primary lesion
         (i.e. 20% of patients with clinically negative
         nodes will have unrecognized metastases)
      b. 60% of patients with unilaterally positive
         lymph nodes will in fact have bilateral
         disease
      c. nodes which appear after removal of the
         primary tumor should be assumed to be
         malignant
      d. 50-75% of patients who subsequently develop

positive lymph nodes can be cured with
lymphadenectomy.
  e. radiation therapy (over 5000 R) will cure only
     20% of patients with proven positive lymph
     nodes
  f. prophylactic irradiation to clinically
     negative nodes has minimal effect.
  g. prophylactic lymphadenectomy has not shown
     improved survival over delayed
     lymphadenectomy.
  h. combined pelvic and radical inguinal lymph
     node dissection has improved prognosis over
     inguinal dissection alone.
  i. no controlled series studying:
     - early vs. delayed lymph node dissection
     - value of radiotherapy or chemotherapy as
     adjunct
2. Recommendations for treatments Stage I and II
  a. bilateral inguinal and pelvic lymph node
     dissection in patients with clinically
     negative nodes when close follow-up will be
     difficult.
  b. delay surgery in reliable and closely followed
     patients and do bilateral pelvic and inguinal
     lymph node dissection if node becomes
     clinically positive.
  c. add radiation therapy over 5000R if concerned
     about margins
  d. ? role of chemotherapy

Stage III

1. Background

  a. untreated --- Zero 5-year survivors
  b. radiation therapy less than half as effective
     as surgery as single modality treatment
  c. 30-60% of patients cured by bilateral pelvic
     and inguinal lymph node dissection.
  d. no controlled studies evaluating adjuvant
     therapy
2. Recommendations for treatment of Stage III
   disease
  a. bilateral pelvic and inguinal lymphadenectomy
     in all patients
  b. chemotherapy can be helpful preoperatively to

control tumor while local infection brought
under control in ulcerating groin lesions
c. radiation therapy useful as postoperative
adjuvant in doses over 5000R

Stage IV

1. Background
   a. less than 10% 5-year survival with any
      treatment
   b. death usually from local/regional disease
2. Recommendations for treatment of Stage IV disease
   a. chemotherapy has a primary role
   b. avoid even palliative surgery unless a tumor
      free local margin is likely or hand is forced
      by potential vascular complications
   c. hemipelvicectomy should be considered in
      carefully selected patients with unilateral
      "inoperable" regional disease

K. 5-Year Survival
   Stage I      over 80%
   Stage II     50-80%
   Stage III    20-50%
   Stage IV     less than 10%

L. Surgical Techniques
   1. penectomy
   2. radical groin dissection (incisions, limits)
   3. use of vascularized pedicle flaps

M. Surgical Complications and Prevention
   1. infection --            antibiotics pre-
                              operatively and
                              peri-operatively
   2. lymphedema --           wrap legs
                              peri-operatively, bedrest
                              and Trendelenberg
                              position
   3. flap necrosis/seroma -- use suction drains +
                              pedicle flaps
   4. hernia --               Cooper's ligament repair
                              + use prolene mesh as
                              needed

5. femoral artery blowout --- cover vessels with
                                Sartorious muscle
6. pulmonary emboli --      prophylactic
                            antiocoagulation

CHAPTER 30B

CHEMOTHERAPY OF PENILE CANCER

Marc B. Garnick

As with other forms of squamous cell carcinoma, carcinoma of the penis responds to certain chemotherapeutic agents such as methotrexate, bleomycin and cis-platinum. Because of the relative rarity of the lesion, the chemotherapeutic experience is limited and is usually employed in patients with end stage disease who have been heavily irradiated. However, several recent reports have documented fairly substantial anti-cancer effects with methotrexate and cis-platinum. The published experience using high dose methotrexate with citrovorum factor rescue indicates that 3 of 9 patients (33%) have achieved meaningful remissions. Our experience at the Sidney Farber Cancer Institute, using high dose methotrexate in 4 patients with loco-regional disease from squamous cell carcinoma of the penis, has indicated an overall response rate of 100%, with 50% of the patients demonstrating complete remissions. The dose in the Farber series is 3 gm/M$^2$ weekly followed by citrovorum factor rescue.

Cis-platinum has also been evaluated. Of 6 adequately treated patients, 3 achieved regressions of disease including one complete remission. The doses used ranged between 1.6 mg/kg and 3 mg/kg or 120 mg/m$^2$, repeated every 3-4 weeks.

These encouraging preliminary results would suggest that optimal strategies should include further evaluation of high dose methotrexate and cis-platinum as single agents. This could hopefully be followed by the use of combination chemo-therapy with methotrexate (in moderate or high doses with "citrovorum factor rescue"), cis-platinum and bleomycin. Indeed, the fact that the disease seems to be responsive to chemotherapy would suggest the use of "adjuvant" therapy in earlier stages of disease including those patients found to have microscopic disease in the lymph nodes.

SUGGESTED REFERENCES

1.  Prout, G.R., Jr. and Garnick, M.B.: Carcinoma of the penis. In: Holland, J.F. and Frei, E. III., eds.: Cancer medicine. Philadelphia: Lea and Febiger, second edition, 1982, pp. 1934-1937.

2.  Garnick, M.B., Skarin, A.T. and Steele, G.D., Jr.: Metastatic carcinoma of the penis: Complete remission after high dose methotrexate chemotherapy. J. Urol. 122:202, 1979.

3.  deKernion, J.B. and Persky, L.: Neoplastic lesions of the penis. In: Skinner, D.G. and deKernion, J.B., eds.: Genitourinary cancer. Philadelphia: WB Saunders Co, 1978, pp. 494-508.

4.  Haile, K. and Delclos, L.: The place of radiation therapy in the treatment of carcinoma of the distal end of the penis. Cancer 45:1980.

5.  Hoppman, H.J. and Fraley, E.E.: Squamous cell carcinoma of the penis - A review. J. Urol. 120:393, 1978.

6.  Ichikawa, T., Nakano, I. and Hirokawa, I.: Bleomycin treatment of the tumors of the penis and scrotum. J. Urol. 102:699, 1969.

7.  Merrin, C.E.: Cancer of the penis. Cancer 45:1973, 1980.

8.  Sklaroff, R.B. and Yagoda, A.: Methotrexate in the treatment of penile carcinoma. Cancer 45:214, 1980.

9.  Sklaroff, R.B., and Yagoda, A.: Cis-diamminedichloride platinum II (DDP) in the treatment of penile carcinoma. Cancer 44:1563, 1979.

CHAPTER 31

EPIDEMIOLOGY OF UROLOGIC CANCERS

Frederick Li

Epidemiologic methods are useful for studies of causes of human cancers, including urologic cancers. The major advantage of epidemiology is the relevance of the data to clinical situations, i.e., the study subjects are patients. The drawback of epidemiology is the inability to perform controlled experiments and the uncertainty inherent in trying to establish causal relationships by observational studies.

BLADDER CANCER

1. Demographic characteristics
   A. sex ratio: 3 males/1 female
   B. rate rises with age
   C. whites greater than blacks
   D. time trends - rising in males
   E. geographic variations within the U.S.
   F. Balkan nephropathy - cancer of the renal pelvis and ureter

2. Occupational causes - latency 20-40 years
   A. dye workers - benzidrine, 2-naphthylamine
   B. rubber workers - aromatic amines
   C. leather workers

3. Tobacco
   A. 2-fold increase in bladder cancer among cigarette smokers
   B. risk increases with amount consumed
   C. possible decreased risk with cessation

   D. multiple primaries of bladder and lung

4. Other causal factors
   A. Schistosoma hematobium (squamous carcinoma)
   B. Thorotrast
   C. radiation
   D. phenacetin
   E. chlornaphazine
   F. coffee, artificial sweeteners


KIDNEY CANCER

   1. Demographic characteristics
      A. sex ratio: 2 males/1 female
      B. time trends and geographic patterns – to be
         defined

   2. Causal factors
      A. tobacco – weak relationship
      B. genetic and familial factors


TESTIS CANCER

   1. Demographic characteristics
      A. age-specific rates trimodal
      B. whites greater than blacks
      C. U.S. incidence doubled in 30 years
      D. rates highest at fertile years

   2. Causal factors
      A. cryptorchism – 20-fold increased risk
      B. familial occurrence
      C. other testicular disorders (?) – atrophy,
         orchitis, diethylstilbesterol (DES)


PROSTATE CANCER

   1. Demographic characteristics
      A. usually after age 60
      B. high frequency of occult disease
      C. more common in U.S. and Western Europe
      D. migration alters rates
      E. higher rates in U.S. Blacks

   2. Causal factors
      A. familial occurrence
      B. ? endocrine/marital factors
      C. ? diet
      D. ? cadmium


PENIS CANCER

   1. Demographic characteristics
      A. rare in U.S. and other industrialized nations
      B. pre-malignant diseases
      C. declining rate in many areas
      D. rates increase with age
      E. social class effect

   2. Causal factors
      A. ? lack of circumcision
      B. ? hygiene
      C. ? viral infections
      D. ? association with cancer of the cervix in female
         partners


SUGGESTED REFERENCES

BLADDER

1. Burbank, F. and Fraumeni, J.F., Jr.: Synthetic sweetener
   consumption and bladder cancer trends in the United
   States. Nature 227:296, 1970.

2. Case, R.A.M. et al.: Tumours of the urinary bladder in
   workmen engaged in the manufacture and use of certain
   dyestuff intermediates in the British chemical industry.
   Br. J. Ind. Med. 11:75, 1954.

3. Cole, P., Hoover, R. and Friedell, G.H.: Occupation and
   cancer of the lower urinary tract. Cancer 29:1250, 1972.

4. Gelfand, M., Weinberg, R.W. and Castle, W.M.: Relation
   between carcinoma of the bladder and infestation with
   Schistosoma haematobium. Lancet 1:1249, 1967.

5.  Kessler I.I. and Clark, J.P.: Saccharin, cyclamate, and
    human bladder cancer. No evidence of an association. JAMA
    240:349, 1978.

6.  Johansson, S. and Wahlquist, L.: Tumours of urinary
    bladder and ureter associated with abuse of
    phenacetin-containing analgesics. Acta Path. Microbiol.
    Scand. 85:768, 1977.

7.  Wynder, E.L. and Goldsmith, R.: The epidemiology of
    bladder cancer. A second look. Cancer 40:1246, 1977.


KIDNEY

1.  Bennington, J.L. and Laubscher, F.A.: Epidemiologic
    studies on carcinoma of the kidney. I. Association of
    renal adenocarcinoma with smoking. Cancer 21:1069, 1968.

2.  Cohen, et al.: Hereditary renal-cell carcinoma associated
    with a chromosomal translocation. N. Engl. J. Med.
    301:592, 1979.

3.  Finger-Kantor, A.L., et al.: Epidemiology of renal cancer
    in Connecticut, 1935-1973. JNCI 57:495, 1976.

4.  Wynder, E.L., Mabuchi, K. and Whitmore, W.F., Jr.:
    Epidemiology of adenocarcinoma of the kidney. JNCI
    53:1619, 1974.


TESTIS

1.  Bibbo, M, et al.: Follow-up study of male and female
    offspring of DES-treated mothers: A preliminary report. J
    Reprod. Med. 15:29, 1975.

2.  Clemmesen, J.: A doubling of morbidity from testis
    carcinoma in Copenhagen: 1943-1962. Acta Path. Microbiol.
    Scan. 72:345, 1968.

3.  Dow, J.A. and Mostofi, F.K.: Testicular tumors following
    orchiopexy. South. Med. J. 60:193, 1967.

4.  Morrison, A.S.: Cryptorchidism, hernia, and cancer of the
    testis. JNCI 56:731, 1976.

5.  Stewart, J.R. and Bagshaw, M.A.: Malignant testicular
    tumors appearing simultaneously in identical twins: A case
    report. Cancer 18:895, 1965.


PROSTATE


1.  Armenian, H.K., et al.: Relation between benign prostatic
    hyperplasia and cancer of the prostate-- a prospective and
    retrospective study. Lancet 2:115, 1974.

2.  Breslow, N., et al.: Latent carcinoma of prostate at
    autopsy in seven areas. Int. J. Cancer 20:680, 1977.

3.  Greenwald, P., et al.: Physical and demographic features
    of men before developing cancer of the prostate. JNCI
    53:341, 1974.

4.  Hutchison, G.B.: Epidemiology of prostatic cancer. Sem.
    Oncol. 3:151, 1976.

5.  Lemen, R.A., et al.: Cancer mortality among cadmium
    production workers. Ann. N.Y. Acad. Sci. 271:273, 1976.

6.  Woolf, C.M.: An investigation of the familial aspects of
    carcinoma of the prostate. Cancer 13:739, 1960.


PENIS


1.  Apt, A.: Circumcision and penile cancer. Acta Med. Scand.
    178:493, 1965.

2.  Boxer, R.J. and Skinner, D.G.: Condylomata acuminata and
    squamous cell carcinoma. Urology 9:72, 1977.

3.  Graham, S., et al.: Genital cancer in wives of penile
    cancer patients. Cancer 44:1870, 1979.

4.  Schrek, R. and Lenowitz, H.: Etiologic factors in
    carcinoma of the penis. Cancer Res. 7:180, 1947.

CHAPTER 32

THE EXPANDING ROLE OF MEDICAL ONCOLOGY IN GENITOURINARY CANCER

Emil Frei, III

Clinical investigative and basic science studies are coming together in a number of areas. These are providing a number of new therapeutic concepts, strategies, and tactics, some of which are currently in clinical trial or will be in the near future. It is the intent of this lecture to cover some of the more representative and promising areas.

NEOADJUVANT CHEMOTHERAPY

Twenty years ago chemotherapy for non-hematologic malignancies was employed only in patients with advanced disease. In the 1970's, well-designed adjuvant studies were performed wherein chemotherapy was delivered immediately followed by surgery and/or radiotherapy (SR). In the past 5 years or less, a number of studies have been introduced wherein treatment is initiated with chemotherapy. There are two major bases for this. 1) To improve local control. For example, in patients with head and neck cancer where chemotherapy is highly effective, albeit remissions are short, such treatment is being employed to reduce the size of the primary such that it is potentially completely controllable by SR. 2) Early treatment of micrometastases. Somatic mutation theory indicates that the development of drug resistant lines and micrometastases may occur in a relatively short period of time (1-2 months) and that pertubation of micrometastases by surgery and/or radiotherapy by altering the coagulation and immunologic system might adversely effect the frequency and rate of growth of micrometastases. For these reasons, several protocols (eg. osteosarcoma) now involve initial treatment

263

with chemotherapy followed later by control of the primary
with SR.  The role of chemotherapy is also evolving in
testicular cancer and possibly (preoperative cisplatin) in
bladder cancer.


MOLECULAR PHARMACOLOGY

     Cisplatin is an effective agent for the treatment of
bladder cancer and shows some activity in combination chemotherapy for the treatment of prostate cancer.  It is the
central drug for the treatment of testicular cancer.  DNA
sequencing studies have allowed us to define at a molecular
level the precise site of breaking and liganding of DNA, and
the relevant repair processes are also under study.  These
studies have guided, to some extent, the synthesis of platinum
analogs, some of which show a lesser nephrotoxicity.
Intercalating substances, such as the anthracyclines, may
influence or direct the site of DNA damage by platinum.  This
may, in part, explain the synergy.  Other organic derivatives
of heavy metals are being prepared that have some degree of
experimental activity and hopefully will be active in GU
cancers.  In short, experimental and clinical studies focusing
on the clinical pharmacology of platinum, combination chemotherapy with platinum, metabolic modulation studies, new
analogs and new clinical treatment strategies deserve major
emphasis.  The use of adriamycin intravesically for superficial bladder cancer and the use of platinum as adjuvant in
patients with invasive bladder cancer deserve emphasis.


DIFFERENTIATION

     There are a number of experiments of nature, including
iatrogenic experiments, that indicate that human tumor cells
are capable of differentiation in vivo.  This includes neuroblastoma, testicular cancer (under the influence of chemotherapy), preleukemia, and a number of additional anecdotal
settings.  Experimentally, it has been possible to induce
differentiation fairly reproducibly in a number of systems.
These include microenvironmental manipulations such as the
mouse embryonal cell carcinoma-hybrid experiments.  Also
experiments that influence the rate of DNA chain elongation
and/or methylation, such as those involving DMSO, Ara-C and
Azacytidine, produce a differentiation in a number of
experimental tumors.  A very interesting "differentiation"

includes analogs of vitamin A which promote differentiation of normal cells as well as abnormal cells experimentally and has been demonstrated to be capable of decreasing the number and magnitude of preneoplastic lesions in the bronchi of smokers. Such agents both at the level of chemo-prevention and chemo-differentiation are currently in early clinical trial.

IMMUNOLOGY

The current revolution in immunology, fueled by monoclonal antibody technology, is already impacting on Phase I strategies. For example, organ-specific antibodies to prostate cancer have been identified which cross-react with many human tumor cells derived from the prostate. Many monoclonal antibodies to various differentiation steps of tissue have been identified, some of which cross-react with neoplastic cells that derive from the relevant early differentiation step. These antibodies, or fragments thereof (FAB), are under study for their diagnostic (labeled with radionuclides) and treatment potential. The antibodies alone may cause cytotoxicity by complement fixation, by activating macrophages, or by inducing antibody dependent cell mediated cytotoxicity. The complexing of these antibodies with highly cytotoxic cancer chemotherapeutic agents and toxins is well along, and such agents are being introduced in clinical trials.

CYTOKINETIC STRATEGIES

There are a number of cytokinetic strategies. One is based on synchronizing hormone-dependent cells. Preliminary studies in patients with receptor-positive breast cancer have indicated that tamoxifen turn-off followed by high dose diethystilbesterol will flux a large cohort of cells into cycle and allow for substantial cytotoxicity with cell-cycle-specific chemotherapeutic agents.

METABOLIC MODULATION

Methotrexate is active in bladder cancer. Methotrexate modulated by Citrovorum Factor Rescue provides the best therapeutic index for choriocarcinoma in women. The metabolic effects of platinum, for example, may be modified by sodium thiosulfate, which concentrates in the urine and prevents, in

experimental animals, the nephrotoxic effect. Almost all of
the antitumor antimetabolites may be modulated biochemically
or pharmacologically by related metabolites, and some of these
strategies have therapeutic potential.


SENSITIZERS

Radiotherapy is an important component of many new
tumors. The nitroimidazole group of compounds have some
activity against hypoxic cells and particularly sensitized
hypoxic cells to radiation by providing a target for free-
radical production. Bioreductive alkylating agents may be
selectively activated by hypoxic cells.


MICROENVIRONMENT ENDOCRINOLOGY

There are a number of hormones or modulators produced in
the micro environment which regulate the behavior of adjacent
cells. These included differentiators, repressors, stimu-
lators of DNA synthesis and protectants such as Interferon.
They also include growth promoters such as nerve growth
factor, all of which modulate normal cells, but neoplastic
cells as well, and many of which can be manipulated by
analogs, by antibodies to receptors, and by manipulation of
cyclic nucleosides.


GENE PRODUCTS

It has been demonstrated by Cooper and Weinberg that human
tumor cells, such as bladder carcinoma, contain DNA which is
capable of transforming normal mouse cells to tumor cells.
Purified DNA is obtained from the human tumor and transferred
into the mouse cell by the calcium precipitate technique.
Using restriction enzyme and other approaches, it is highly
likely that the specific gene or set of genes responsible for
such transformation will be identified in relatively near
future. In addition, specific gene products, such as p60 SRC,
will be identified. Two therapeutic approaches include 1)
control of transforming gene activity by a DNA sequence with
some homology to the transforming gene, and 2) transition
state analogs to the 60SRC which has protein kinase activity,
particularly for the cytoskeleton.

These are only a few of some of the exciting new approaches to the treatment of GU cancer which are in early clinical trial today or will be in the relatively near future.

SELECTED REFERENCES

1.  Frei, E. III and Ervin, T.J.: Summary and overview. In: Salmon, S.E. and Jones, S.E. eds.: Adjuvant Therapy of Cancer. New York: Grune and Stratton, 1981, p. 569.

2.  Goldie, J.H. and Coldman, A. J. A mathematical model for relating drug sensitivity of tumors to their spontaneous mutation rate. Cancer Treat. Rep. 63:1727, 1979.

3.  Prestayko, A.W., Crooke, S.T. and Carter, S.K. eds. Cisplatin: Current status and new developments. New York: Academic Press, 1980.

4.  Ruddon, R.W., Cancer Biology. Oxford University Press, 1981, p. 99.

5.  Reinherz, E.L., et al. Discrete stages of intrathymic differentiation: analysis of normal thymocyles and leukemic lymphoblastis of T-lineage. Proc. Natl. Acad. Sci. 77:1588, 1980.

CONTRIBUTORS

WILLIAM D. BLOOMER, M.D.
Assistant Professor of Radiation Therapy
Harvard Medical School
Radiation Therapist
Sidney Farber Cancer Institute
Boston, Massachusetts

Chapter 25 - Radiation Therapy Complications of the
Genitourinary Tract

LESLIE BOTNICK, M.D.
Assistant Professor of Radiation Therapy
Harvard Medical School
Radiation Therapist
Beth Israel Hospital
Boston, Massachusetts

Chapter 8 - The Role of Radiation Therapy in Renal
Carcinoma

GEORGE P. CANELLOS, M.D.
Associate Professor of Medicine
Harvard Medical School
Chief, Division of Medical Oncology
Sidney Farber Cancer Institute
Associate Physician in Medicine
Brigham and Women's Hospital
Boston, Massachusetts

Chapter 9 - Management of Isolated Metastases and
Advanced Renal Cell Cancer

J. ROBERT CASSADY, M.D.
Associate Professor of Radiation Therapy
Harvard Medical School
Senior Associate in Radiation Therapy
Joint Center for Radiation Therapy
Boston, Massachusetts

Chapter 4 - External Beam Irradiation for Carcinoma of the Prostate

Chapter 11A - Wilms' Tumor - Natural History

LAWRENCE H. EINHORN, M.D.
Professor of Medicine
Indiana University Medical School
Indianapolis, Indiana

Chapter 16 - Systemic Chemotherapy in the Management of Bladder Cancer

Chapter 18 - Chemotherapy of Testis Cancer

JUDAH FOLKMAN, M.D.
Julia Dyckman Andrus Professor of Pediatric Surgery and Professor of Anatomy
Harvard Medical School
Senior Associate in Surgery
Children's Hospital Medical Center
Boston, Massachusetts

Chapter 11B - Wilms' Tumor - Surgical Aspects

EMIL FREI III, M.D.
Professor of Medicine
Harvard Medical School
Director and Physician-in-Chief
Sidney Farber Cancer Institute
Boston, Massachusetts

Chapter 32 - The Expanding Role of Medical Oncology in Genitourinary Cancer

MARC B. GARNICK, M.D.
Assistant Professor of Medicine
Harvard Medical School
Assistant Physician
Sidney Farber Cancer Institute
Attending Physician in Medicine
Brigham and Women's Hospital
Boston, Massachusetts

Chapter 5 - Management of Advanced Prostate Cancer

Chapter 6 - Renal Cell Carcinoma - Diagnostic Workup
    and Natural History

Chapter 10 - Cancers of the Renal Pelvis and Ureter

Chapter 13 - Intravesical Chemotherapy for Superficial
    Bladder Carcinoma

Chapter 23 - Assessment of Renal Function II - Cancer
    Chemotherapy Induced Nephrotoxicity

Chapter 30B - Chemotherapy of Penile Cancer

SAMUEL HELLMAN, M.D.
    Alvin T. & Viola D. Fuller, American Cancer Society
    Professor and Chairman of Radiation Therapy
    Harvard Medical School
    Director, Joint Center for Radiation Therapy
    Boston, Massachusetts

    Chapter 15 - Radiation Therapy in the Management of
        Bladder Cancer

WILLIAM D. KAPLAN, M.D.
    Associate Professor of Radiology
    Harvard Medical School
    Chief, Oncologic Nuclear Medicine
    Sidney Farber Cancer Institute
    Boston, Massachusetts

    Chapter 26 - New Diagnostic Techniques
        Lymphoscintigraphy

GARY P. KEARNEY, M.D.
    Clinical Assistant Professor of Surgery (Urology)
    Harvard Medical School
    Associate in Surgery
    Brigham and Women's Hospital
    Boston, Massachusetts

    Chapter 24 - Urologic Complications of Gynecologic
        Cancers

LESTER KLEIN, M.D.
   Associate Professor of Surgery
   Harvard Medical School
   Head, Division of Urology
   Beth Israel Hospital
   Boston, Massachusetts

   Chapter 2 - Surgical Management of Prostate Cancer

FREDERICK LI, M.D.
   Associate Professor of Medicine
   Harvard Medical School
   Associate Physician
   Sidney Farber Cancer Institute
   Boston, Massachusetts

   Chapter 31 - Epidemiology of Urologic Cancers

ALAN B. RETIK, M.D.
   Professor of Surgery
   Harvard Medical School
   Chief, Division of Urology
   Children's Hospital Medical Center
   Boston, Massachusetts

   Chapter 17 - Rhabdomyosarcoma of the Bladder and
      Prostate

JEROME P. RICHIE, M.D.
   Associate Professor of Urologic Surgery
   Harvard Medical School
   Chief of Urologic Oncology
   Brigham and Women's Hospital
   Boston, Massachusetts

   Chapter 6 - Renal Cell Carcinoma - Diagnostic Workup and
      Natural History

   Chapter 7 - Surgical Management of Renal Cell Carcinoma

   Chapter 10 - Cancers of the Renal Pelvis and Ureter

   Chapter 14 - Role of Surgery for Bladder Cancer

   Chapter 19 - Role of Surgery in Early Stage Testis
      Cancer

Chapter 20 - Role of Tumor Reductive Surgery after
Chemotherapy for Testis Cancer

Chapter 29 - Carcinoma of the Adrenal Cortex

RICHARD E. RIESELBACH, M.D.
Professor and Chairman
Department of Medicine
Milwaukee Clinical Campus
University of Wisconsin Medical School
Physician-in-Chief
Department of Medicine
Mount Sinai Medical Center
Milwaukee, Wisconsin

Chapter 22 - Assessment of Renal Function I
Antibiotic Nephrotoxicity in the Patient with
Urologic Cancer

STEPHEN E. SALLAN, M.D.
Associate Professor of Pediatrics
Harvard Medical School
Clinical Director, Pediatric Oncology
Sidney Farber Cancer Institute
Boston, Massachusetts

Chapter 11C - Wilms' Tumor - Chemotherapy

WILLIAM U. SHIPLEY, M.D.
Associate Professor of Radiation Therapy
Harvard Medical School
Radiation Therapist
Massachusetts General Hospital
Boston, Massachusetts

Chapter 3 - Interstitial Radiation Therapy for
Management of Localized Prostate Cancer

DONALD G. SKINNER, M.D.
Professor and Chief
Division of Urology
University of Southern California
School of Medicine
Los Angeles, California

Chapter 14 - Role of Surgery for Bladder Cancer

Chapter 19 - Role of Surgery in Early Stage Testis
    Cancer

Chapter 28 - In Vitro Clonogenic Chemosensitivity Assay
    in Urologic Tumors

RALPH R. WEICHSELBAUM, M.D.
    Associate Professor of Radiation Therapy
    Harvard Medical School
    Associate in Radiation Therapy
    Joint Center for Radiation Therapy
    Boston, Massachusetts

    Chapter 21 - Seminoma

WILLET F. WHITMORE JR., M.D.
    Professor of Surgery
    Cornell Medical School
    Chief, Division of Urology
    Memorial Sloan-Kettering Cancer Center
    New York, New York

    Chapter 1 - Prostate Cancer - Natural History and
        Staging

WILLET F. WHITMORE III, M.D.
    Assistant Professor in Urologic Surgery
    Harvard Medical School
    Surgeon, Division of Urology
    Brigham and Women's Hospital
    Boston, Massachusetts

    Chapter 30A - Carcinoma of the Penis

BRUCE R. ZETTER, Ph.D.
    Assistant Professor of Microbiology and
    Molecular Genetics in the Department of Surgery
    Harvard Medical School
    Research Associate
    Children's Hospital Medical Center
    Boston, Massachusetts

    Chapter 27 - A New Marker for the Detection of
        Transitional Cell Carcinoma

LEONARD N. ZINMAN, M.D.
    Clinical Assistant Professor in Surgery
    Harvard Medical School
    Urologic Consultant
    Lahey Clinic Medical Center
    Boston, Massachusetts

    Chapter 12 - Bladder Cancer - Natural History